Users' Voices

The perspectives of mental health service users on community and hospital care

Diana Rose

Photography: Jon Walter

ISBN: 1 870480 47 3

Published by

The Sainsbury Centre for Mental Health
134-138 Borough High Street
London
SE1 1LB

Tel: 020 7403 8790
Fax: 020 7403 9482

www.sainsburycentre.org.uk

The Sainsbury Centre for Mental Health is a registered charity, working to improve the quality of life for people with severe mental health problems. It aims to influence national policy and encourage good practice in mental health services, through a co-ordinated programme of research, training and development. The Centre is affiliated to King's College London (School of Health and Life Sciences).

Charity registration number 291308

ACKNOWLEDGEMENTS

The Sainsbury Centre for Mental Health has a tradition of involving users in research and evaluation. The beginnings of User-Focused Monitoring (UFM) lay in negotiations between Kensington & Chelsea and Westminster (KCW) Health Authority and the Centre, when Matt Muijen and Richard Ford proposed that evaluation of the CPA would include users interviewing a large sample of other users from the top tier of the CPA. UFM as a model and a method was developed and implemented by Diana Rose with the KCW UFM user group. Libby Gawith helped with the questionnaire design and Peter Lindley developed the training model. UFM was deployed in subsequent sites by Brigid Morris, Gabriel Mackintosh, Jim Green, Jeanette Copperman and Nutan Kotecha. Thanks also to Kerry O'Mahoney, Shirley Morrison and Siân Taylder for doing mountains of photocopying and dealing with hundreds of letters and telephone calls.

CONTENTS

Background

User-Focused Monitoring (UFM) was first developed and pioneered by the Sainsbury Centre for Mental Health in 1997 with a pilot user-run project in the London Borough of Kensington & Chelsea and Westminster (KCW).

The main purpose of UFM is systematically to find out what mental health service users think about living in the community, of their services and of their experiences of being in hospital.

This report is, of course, not the first time user views have been represented, but it is perhaps the first time mental health service users with severe and enduring mental health problems (i.e. in regular contact with mental health services) have created, developed carried out and analysed such a major piece of research. Some 61 user interviewers were trained and carried out the eight projects which make up this report. They interviewed over 500 service users living both in the community, and in hospital on seven sites situated in urban, rural and seaside areas of England.

The fact that the questions were developed and asked by user interviewers is important and affected the interviewee's responses. The interviewers reported back that service users visibly relaxed and opened up once they knew the interviewer had also 'been through the system' and understood their own situation.

Aims

Users' Voices is not only an important report because of the groundbreaking way in which the research was undertaken, but for what it aims to achieve – which is to represent service users who often do not have a voice, or if they do it is not heard.

The report produced from the KCW project (D. Rose *et al.,* 1998) showed that people with mental health problems are perfectly capable of judging the services they receive, of praising where praise is due and making balanced criticisms when they don't. *Users' Voices* now takes that work further and proves, by pulling together user's experiences in seven different sites, that their views of services are consistent and cohesive.

The audience

The report is aimed at a diverse audience of mental health service planners and managers, policy makers, service users, practitioners and researchers.

Political context

According to health secretary Alan Milburn, 'The patient is king'. This is excellent news for the patient with a physical illness, but this report shows that it is still unclear to mental health service users whether this kingship includes them. However, Milburn's words at least express an encouraging intention. Additionally, the NHS Plan for a patient centred health service and other government legislation puts the patient/service user at the centre of his or her care – at least on paper.

The research

Users' Voices is a unique report in many ways not least because the research questions were developed by users and were very different to those usually found in professional research questionnaires. The researchers were keen to find out users' views on a range of different topics – though all related to their use of mental health services. There were variations in the questionnaires according to each site's specific remit and these are highlighted in the report, but there were also some core questions which were asked on all sites.

The fact that the interviewers were all service users themselves made a huge difference. As the introduction to the report points out they were not the 'worried well', some of them were on the top tier of the CPA. And yet with the right training all completed their interviews and all gained in confidence as a result of doing so. More than that they realised that they were gaining a different and more open response from their interviewees than professional researchers might have done.

The UFM interviewers worked in seven sites, which ranged from inner city London to comparatively rural Huntingdon (Cambridgeshire) and the northern seaside town of Scarborough (Yorkshire). Interviewers visited service users in their own homes, in supported housing and in hospital.

These service users received a range of different types of mental health services, delivered by a range of mental health professionals who included community support workers, community psychiatric nurses (CPNs) and social workers. The majority of the interviewees had severe and enduring mental health problems, were on medication and most were on the top tier of the CPA (representing a high level of need).

The sites visited included a health authority, a trust, a social services department and a voluntary agency. All were progressive in their approach (which can be seen from the fact that they had commissioned UFM in the first place) and their commissioners had a commitment to how users viewed their services. However, despite this commitment, interviewers encountered some reticence and even resistance to the research on the part of some frontline staff.

The core questions

Although UFM questionnaires were tailor-made to fulfil the specific brief they had for each site, they all included questions that covered the key areas of:

* information
* the care delivery process
* clinical issues
* mental health crises

* user involvement
* advocacy, health records and complaints
* user satisfaction with care.

The findings

Information

Mental health service users need information to make informed choices about their care. Around 50 % of users interviewed for this work felt they were not getting enough information on a range of issues and therefore felt themselves to be recipients of rather than involved in their mental health care. The report's overall findings show that access to good information is significantly associated with how satisfied users say they are with mental health services as a whole.

Care delivery

The care programme approach (CPA) is what governs the care of people with mental health problems living in the community. However, this report found that the majority of service users do not know what the CPA is for. Government policy is that users should be involved in drawing up their care plan (DoH 1999). But of all the sites visited by UFM interviewers only service users in Huntingdon even knew who their CPA key workers were or that they had a care plan. Even fewer service users knew the date of their next CPA review.

Clinical issues

Clinical issues cover the forms of help available for service users from psychiatric services. They provide a focus around which UFM and processional research can be compared. Mental health professionals assess service users according to their 'needs'. This report suggests that these needs are sometimes interpreted as 'problems'. Most service users felt their strengths and abilities had not been considered.

Medication

While many users suffered from the side effects of psychotropic drugs, most also appreciated the benefits and lessening of symptoms. It was also clear that black service users were more likely to receive medication by injection than white service users – particularly if male.

Someone to talk to

When asked what was missing from their care a large number of users said 'someone to talk to'. Although talking therapies were popular amongst users that had access to them what many seemed to want was 'a sympathetic ear' and the chance to talk about ordinary things.

Mental health crises

A mental health crisis will disrupt a service user's life and that of their family/carers. Where service users have to be admitted to hospital and/or detained under the Mental Health Act the situation is particularly traumatic.

Despite the gravity of these types of situations, not all interviewees knew who to contact in a crisis.

Discharge procedures

The hospital discharge process, if handled ineptly or mistimed, can have disastrous consequences for the service user. The 1999 *Confidential Inquiry into Homicides and Suicides by Mentally Ill People* found that most suicides occurred in the week following discharge from hospital. However, despite these well-documented findings, this report shows that users' perceptions of discharge are still not positive.

User involvement

This report shows conclusively that users still do not feel involved in making decisions about their care at any level. It is clear that the government's intention of putting the patient 'at the centre' has not filtered down to all those who provide mental health services – be they organisations or individual mental health professionals.

Advocacy, health records and complaints

A service user's access to advocacy, health records and a complaints system can all contribute to a greater sense of involvement in his or mental health care and are interconnected. The report's findings suggest that while users knew about these procedures they do not access them.

User satisfaction

There were marked differences in user satisfaction with professionals between those who lived in rural and inner city areas, especially in terms of medical staff.

In a general question relating to overall user satisfaction there was no evidence of what researchers call the 'halo' effect – (a term given to exaggerated satisfaction ratings on standard questionnaires). It seems that by asking a range of questions related to the subject, UFM interviewers gained fuller and therefore less glowing responses from service users. The report suggests that user responses depend very much on the questions put.

The future

A follow-up review of the KCW site shows that User-Focused Monitoring can make a difference to the lives of service users. Staff had initiated many changes as a result of the first project's findings and these had clearly taken effect.

Many of the interviewers found that they gained substantially from the process in terms of enhanced self-esteem. Some are now in full time employment, while others have set up as consultants in user-focused research.

Now UFM is set to move into the field of service development – by enabling other service users to participate in user-led evaluations within their own areas. The aim is to concentrate on solutions rather than problems and to ensure that the concerns raised in *Users' Voices* are effectively addressed as services evolve.

In conclusion, *Users' Voices* proves categorically, against a background of solid methodology and analysis, that mental health services users not only have something to say about the services they receive but that what they say is sound, rational and can be taken on its own merits.

The report begins with a set of strong recommendations and concludes with a set of user-defined standards for good mental health care (see questionnaires in Appendices C and D) which if taken together will help take user-focused mental health care off the research page and into practice.

KEY RECOMMENDATIONS

GENERAL

- Users should be involved in training all psychiatric and social care professionals. User training should be built into the curricula for psychiatrists, psychiatric nurses, social workers and occupational therapists. Such training should aim to give mental health professionals a detailed understanding of the experience of using services and the implications of this experience for professional practice.

- Users should be involved in training the police both broadly and specifically in relation to mental health crises. The police should understand that being in a crisis does not mean that users are unaware of how they are being treated with regard to physical force, respect and dignity.

- Mental health and associated professionals should change their focus from a 'problems' model of their clients to a fully developed 'strengths' model. Professionals should develop care in line with users' self-definition of their needs and should build on users' strengths in a way that involves service users at all levels of care.

- Inpatient units should not be allowed to deteriorate further as alternatives to inpatient care are put in place. Inpatient units should be a priority for environmental and therapeutic improvement.

SPECIFIC

- All prescriptions for psychotropic medication, including prescriptions from hospital pharmacies, should provide full information on the benefits and side effects of the drugs. Inpatient units should hold this information in accessible leaflet form for all the medications used on the ward.

- Non-medical staff who take on the keyworking role, such as social workers and occupational therapists, should be trained in the main side effects of common psychiatric drugs.

- CMHTs should develop central, indexed, stores of information concerning community resources, housing, benefits, work projects and advocacy. All staff should have a basic knowledge of what these stores contain. Inpatient units should have freely available leaflets on the main resources in their locality. This information should be available in all the locally spoken languages and in forms accessible to those with sensory impairments.

- Purchasers and providers should facilitate, but not control, user involvement and empowerment at all levels from individual care through service management to service planning, by providing resources, including finance, and training and by making planning and management procedures transparent and accessible.

- User involvement in planning and delivering individual care should be for purposes of empowerment not compliance.

- The measurement of the extent of user involvement at all levels should be the extent to which users themselves feel involved.

- The complaints of users should be taken seriously. They must not be pathologised or dismissed as symptoms of mental illness and those who complain should not feel they are being branded as trouble makers or fear repercussions.

- There should be a systematic, user-led evaluation of models of advocacy in mental health in the UK.

- Users should be at the centre of the monitoring and evaluation of mental health services.

PART I

USER-FOCUSED

MONITORING

THE MODEL

AND

THE METHOD

INTRODUCTION

This report introduces a model and a method for evaluating and researching the experiences of mental health service users in community and hospital settings. The model has service users at its core. An initial study has already been published (Rose *et al.*, 1998). The report covers projects carried out between 1996 and 1999. It is the final statement on the first phase of the work. Since then, the method has developed and new findings have emerged. These developments will soon be available on CD-ROM and the Internet.

Three large claims are made for our approach. It empowers service users by giving them real work as interviewers. It enables the voices of the most disabled users to be both heard and have an influence on care delivery. And, finally, it provides more accurate and sensitive information about users' experiences of mental health services than do traditional, professional approaches. The approach is known as User-Focused Monitoring or UFM and it has been developed and implemented at the Sainsbury Centre for Mental Health (SCMH) over the past four years.

The bulk of this report is a presentation and discussion of the results of interviews, site visits and a focus group. Over 500 mental health service users participated in this research. Most of these had severe and enduring mental health problems. In this introduction, we summarise the model and the method. In chapter 2, we look at the process of putting the model into practice. Chapter 3 consists of a series of unedited accounts written by users who participated as interviewers in our research. Part 2 describes the groups of users interviewed and contains a detailed presentation and discussion of what these users told us about the mental health services they were receiving. Part 3 comprises a commentary on the findings. There are four Appendices: one methodological, one statistical and two lists of questions which can also be framed as standards for good mental health care. Appendix C lists questions used in the community research and Appendix D lists questions asked during site visits to acute units.

UFM – The Principles

UFM is user-focused in at least five ways.

* Most of the people working centrally to co-ordinate research and evaluation are users or former users of psychiatric services.

* The instruments used are constructed by groups of local service users. Whilst those working centrally also have professional qualifications, the local service users are in touch with grass roots services.

* These local service users also carry out the practical research work: one-to-one interviews, site visits and focus groups.

* Our informants are people who make heavy use of psychiatric services. Usually, they are users with severe and enduring mental health problems and as such they are often denied a voice.

* Finally, results are interpreted and reports written from the service user's perspective, that is, through the eyes of the project co-ordinators.

The aim of UFM is to evaluate mental health provision from the perspectives of service users with severe and enduring mental health problems. UFM as a model and a method has been developed so that these perspectives are accurately portrayed.

Chapter 2 shows in detail how these principles are put into practice in research and evaluation work.

UFM so far

So far, UFM has trained and supported 61 user researchers. Some of these have gone on to find full-time work and some have continued with other UFM or associated projects. There are also 17 users currently being trained for UFM projects.

By the beginning of 2000, we had interviewed more than 500 service users most of whom had severe and enduring mental health problems. This includes users interviewed on a one-to-one basis, most of whom were living in the community, and users interviewed during site visits, most of whom were in acute hospitals or day hospitals. We believe that this database is unique both in size and in detail.

Outcomes

Part of the purpose of UFM is systematically to find out what mental health service users think about living in the community, their experiences with particular services or particular groups of workers, or their experiences of being in hospital. We would argue that, with a few exceptions, such work is in its infancy. We also argue for its importance because, until recently, mental health service users have not had a voice either in research and evaluation or in influencing care delivery.

In an era where we hear much about social exclusion, stigmatisation and empowerment, it is vital to listen to the voices of those who are excluded, stigmatised and disempowered.

But UFM always started with more modest aims. Each of the projects to be reported here was commissioned by a specific agency – a health authority, a trust, a social services department or a voluntary agency. These agencies sought to find out how their particular services were viewed by the people who were the recipients. The agencies that sought these views were not a random selection. They saw themselves as in the forefront of the movement to empower mental health service users and they believed that UFM could identify gaps in their services which they could take steps to remedy. Indeed, we shall see later that with the longitudinal evaluation this belief bore fruit. The sites where we worked all incorporated our findings into their mental health strategies, and one at least now bases its mental health performance targets on the findings of UFM.

UFM has its limitations. Because it was commissioned by agencies providing mental health services, its focus is on these services. We are well aware that contact with mental health services does not exhaust users' experiences of living in the community. It will be seen that community services are very broadly defined in UFM. At the same time, it is important to note that some of the people who participated in these studies were living very isolated lives in the community. On more than a few occasions, we visited people who had no local contacts bar the home help that did their weekly shop and their keyworker. They had left the old institutions only to be ghettoised in the community. Stigma and social exclusion were a daily part of their lives. For these users, and for many others we talked to, mental health *services* were critical to their quality of life, for good or ill.

THE PROCESS

In this chapter, we seek to be as explicit as possible about the process of UFM research or evaluation. This is so that the reader can readily interrogate our method and come to their own conclusion as to how robust it is. At the same time, we would like readers to be able to use this chapter to carry out UFM themselves. Those interested in the more academic aspects of methodology in relation to UFM are referred to Appendix A.

We should say at the outset that in some respects our approach is very traditional. It uses the tried and tested social research methods of questionnaire design, interviewing, processing the results through a computer package and producing an analysis. However, users are central to each step of the process in UFM and this is what makes the approach different to more orthodox ones in social research. We shall see as we proceed that there are consequent changes to the research process as such.

Groundwork

The key to any piece of UFM work is a local group of service users. Working with UFM groups is always a lively and challenging experience. Each project has its own group. The first step for the project co-ordinator is to recruit group members. This involves going to day centres, work projects and so on and explaining the project. Some people in these settings are immediately keen to be involved. At the same time, we are often met with many that lack self-confidence. A majority of users in these initial talks think the project will be too difficult for them. Overcoming this lack of self-confidence is a task that continues throughout the life of the project. We have come to the conclusion that mental health services are very good at telling people what they *cannot* do. On a more positive note, it is almost always the case that those who begin the project go on to complete their work.

Those who have been persuaded to give UFM a try come to a lunchtime meeting over sandwiches and tea and coffee. We go into the project in some more detail. But much of the first meeting is always spent reassuring people that if we can do it, so can they; after all we are service users too. We say that we will support them throughout the project and that they will always be free to turn things down. But we also make it plain that what they will be doing is real work and that they will be paid the same rate that we pay other researchers. The members of the group should now be in a position to decide whether they want to continue with the project.

UFM groups meet fortnightly or monthly, depending on the project timetable. The first three or four meetings are spent constructing a questionnaire, site visit workbook or set of focus group questions. These meetings are vital because they are the means of ensuring that the instruments are firmly rooted in users' experiences of community and hospital services. This method of generating user-defined instruments distinguishes UFM as a method from research designed by professionals. We will show in the following chapters how it also generates a different picture of mental health services from that painted by professional research.

It should not be thought that these meetings are quiet, subdued affairs. They are argumentative and full of conflict as the lack of self-confidence evident earlier gradually evaporates. People come to see that they are indeed experts in mental health care and they come to want their experience represented in the instruments.

Developing the questionnaire

Usually, the project co-ordinator will bring a skeleton tool to the first of these meetings. For the first group, convened in Kensington & Chelsea and Westminster Health Authority (see chapter 5) this skeleton tool was very sketchy indeed. The group worked very hard to construct a full community care questionnaire and it was this tool that subsequent groups were presented with in the first instance. The subsequent groups made many changes to the development group's questionnaire to tailor it to their specific project. However, there are a set of 'core questions' which most groups retained and it is these which we will use to present our findings in Part 2. These core questions are listed in Appendix C. The user groups compiled a parallel set of questions for acute units and these can be found in Appendix D.

Faced with the development tool, the group is free to start again from scratch if they wish. One group did so. More often, they worked with the tool but amended it heavily, deleted and added questions and crossed and re-crossed out wordings. At the end of the meeting, the project co-ordinator has the task of producing a new version taking into account all that has been said at the meeting. This process has to be gone through three or four times until the whole group is happy with what has been produced. There is one final chance to re-draft and that is at the pilot stage.

The kinds of question generated by UFM groups look very different to those usually found in professional questionnaires. Firstly, the questions tend to cover a much broader range of issues than traditional tools. But even where the topics covered are similar, user groups generate different types of question to those found in professional scales. For instance, professional interviews, like UFM interviews, often ask about medication. But professional interviews tend to focus on issues of compliance whereas UFM groups design questions asking about choice, dignity, information about side effects and respect. UFM questions are also very detailed and specific. For example, UFM groups do not just consider medication in a different light to professionals, they want to know exactly what it is about taking medication that users like and do not like.

Training

The next stage in the life of a UFM user group is training. Again, this was slightly different for the first group than subsequent ones. The development project did not start training until the questionnaire had been completed. In some subsequent groups, because the 'skeleton' tool was fuller, questionnaire design and training took place concurrently.

The time training takes depends on the technique used. It takes much longer to train a group in one-to-one interviewing with a complex schedule than it does to train in site visiting. Of course, all techniques have the advantage that the group has constructed the tool itself and so is thoroughly familiar with it.

For complex schedules, some instruction is necessary in how to fill them out to correspond with the interviewees' answers. It should be remembered that nearly all of our user researchers are new to this task. Many mistakes are made and frustration is evident. However, the training must be successful because all the completed schedules have been properly filled out.

Role-play is the main method of training. There are of course serious reasons for this. It is important that interviewers learn to take the role of the interviewee and discover what it is like to be on the receiving end of the questions. In this way, they learn what sense a question makes or does not make if asked in a certain way and they also learn how to pace themselves with different interviewees. The serious dimension of role-play is obviously important but it is also important that the whole process is fun. Often the atmosphere is hilarious and is crucial for building self-confidence and providing a social glue for the group.

By this time, our groups of timid users are usually transformed into confident, competent interviewers and ready to go. They have one last task and this is to carry out a pilot. We arrange for the group to go to a setting where there are mental health service users similar to those they are going to interview. Each user interviewer is paired with a volunteer interviewee who is paid for their time. The interviewer takes them through the questions. The co-ordinator moves between the pairs noting down any final tips for the interviewers. S/he collects the completed schedules and goes through them for any final problems. The next time the group meets, they de-brief on the pilot and usually the interviewers are both very pleased with their performance and a little awed at what is to come.

Obstacles

However, before the interviewers can move into the real world, the co-ordinator faces some very different obstacles. Whilst the training is going on, s/he has to find a suitable group of interviewees. This requires co-ordination with purchasers and providers.

UFM chooses its interviewees by means of random sampling partly because this is a means of ensuring that everyone has the chance to be included, including people who are very isolated. Details can be found in Appendix A. However, choosing the interviewees is only the first step.

Next we have to contact them to see if they are willing to be interviewed. We do this by letter via their keyworker, as we cannot have access to their addresses for reasons of confidentiality.

It rapidly became clear when we started UFM that not all keyworkers passed the letters on. Most who did not, said they were too busy and it was not a priority. However, some were actively hostile to the idea of users interviewing users or did not believe their clients could give valid answers to the questions. Indeed, one psychotherapist explicitly said that his client's criticisms of services were a "symptom of her psychopathology".

It has to be remembered that the sites in which we worked had all commissioned UFM which was a novel and relatively untried approach. The commissioners, at least, were committed to finding out users' views. We had more trouble with frontline staff some of whom seemed to hold traditional views of mental distress. We might have had even more trouble in sites with less progressive commissioners and this does not bode well for any policy initiative which seeks to empower mental health service users. However, this type of resistance has decreased with time.

There tended to be two consequences of the patchy contact we made with potential interviewees. First, our final response rates were relatively disappointing although they were no lower than those found in comparable research (see Appendix A). Secondly, the interviews we carried out in community sites tended to be stretched out over an extended period of time as we made wave after wave of attempt to persuade keyworkers to pass on letters. The final thing to be said about this aspect of the research is that setting up the interviews is always a bureaucratic nightmare. Matching interviewer and interviewee and finding mutually convenient venues, times and dates as well as being available to de-brief an interviewer immediately after an interview should not be underestimated by anyone who would like to carry out work like this.

The interviewers' experiences

So, how did it go? What did we, as co-ordinators, hear back from our interviewers? Often they were delighted to have completed the task successfully. Sometimes they were shocked by the isolation of the people they interviewed. A few have been worried that their interviewee needed something more from them. Often they told of sharing their own experience at the end of the interview. Some were worried that the interview had taken too long because the interviewee had wanted so much to talk. And on three occasions, they asked us to contact a mental health professional so distressed did their interviewee appear. However, in talking to over 500 users, only once did an interviewer come back and say that the interview had been impossible because of the mental state of the user.

The situation with site visits is a little different. First, there are fewer questions (see Appendix D) and the interviews are much shorter. Two members of a user group, accompanied by the project co-ordinator, conduct a site visit, which may be to an acute ward, an intensive care ward, a day hospital or a work project. The user interviewers talk to as many people on the ward or project as are willing to be interviewed.

We believe that we ask quite a lot of our UFM interviewers. They are asked to put their 'selves' into the interview in a way that does not often happen except perhaps with participant observation research. However, as the next chapter will show, we have to conclude that they think it is worthwhile and that they enjoy it. User interviewers never tire of telling us how, at the beginning of a project, they could never have believed that they could do what they end up routinely doing. Without being presumptuous, we think there is a lesson here. Our interviewers are not the so-called 'worried well'. Half of them are on the top tier of the CPA. If they can be trained and supported to do this work and their confidence can be built in the process, so can others.

There is another issue. Early literature on consumer satisfaction with mental health services (Carlsmith and Aronson, 1963) questioned whether mental patients could sensibly make judgements about the quality of services. Although this is no longer said in the research literature, we have seen that the view is evident amongst some of the frontline staff we contact. The experience of our interviewers contradicts this view. The impression we get from our interviewers' accounts is of people willing to share their experience, giving balanced and sound judgements, even of being often denied a listening ear and wanting to sustain the company of the interviewer. This impression will be confirmed often in the findings which follow.

In the methodological appendix (A), we present evidence that user interviewers gain more valid information than professional ones. Our interviewees seemed especially willing to talk to another user, someone who shared their experience and could ask them meaningful questions. It is for these reasons that we argue that a user-focused approach such as this can gather information that is denied to more orthodox research.

The user groups continue to meet as the work proceeds. The purpose of the meetings is to provide opportunities for feedback, mutual support and reassurance and learning from each other. These meetings are usually unstructured, sociable and very noisy! We encourage the user interviewers and site visitors to write about their experience as a contribution to our final reports. Some of these contributions are reprinted in the next section.

The results

Once the data is in, it is the job of the project co-ordinators to analyse it. However, even at this stage, the user groups have a role. For example, one user group member completed the quantitative data input for two projects. And as the analysis proceeds, results are taken back to the group to see how far they correspond with members' impressions of the interviews and site visits.

In this report, we present both quantitative and qualitative findings. The interview results take the form of percentages of respondents endorsing particular questions. We also carry out some further statistical analyses with some of the questions that seemed to be of particular importance. These analyses were carried out using the statistical package SPSS for Windows Version 8. They could be carried out with alternative packages.

The results of the site visits are qualitative. Users fill out site visit workbooks at the end of the visit based on the questions reproduced in Appendix D. There is space for the interviewer's observations and the respondents' comments. These site visit workbooks are summarised and tabulated according to positive findings, problems and recommendations for each topic. The tabulations are checked with the users who carried out the visit. The presentation of results of the site visits will be discursive.

A unique perspective

We believe that all research comes from particular conceptual and ethical standpoints. No research is neutral. Our standpoint in this report is that of the mental health service user. As we have emphasised throughout this chapter, the user's perspective is present in UFM at every stage. This is true also in the writing of this report and in the presentation of results.

The data we analyse and present to the reader is the end-point of a long user-focused process just as any data is the end-point of a long process. We want to reflect what our interviewees said as accurately as possible in what we write and be as true as possible to our informants' views. However, that 'truth' will not spring fully formed from the interview protocols and site visit workbooks. Somebody needs to make sense of the figures and quotes. In UFM, we do this drawing on our own experience as service users. In addition, in this report, we shall be drawing on experience in the UK users' movement and literature from that movement. In case any reader thinks that this amounts to bias, let it be said that we are only being explicit about what happens in all research but which is often left unsaid. Often the 'standpoint' in research is called the 'theory' or the 'conceptual framework'. These are all means of organising and interpreting data and it is important to be explicit about them.

There is one further point to be made about the user-focused nature of the following chapters. Recently, Bauer, Gaskell and Allum (2000) have argued that all research has a rhetorical function. That is, it seeks to persuade an audience of something. Once again, this usually is not acknowledged because it looks suspiciously like 'bias'. But if these authors are right that this function is intrinsic to research writing, we are not shy of saying that in this report we seek to persuade. We want our readers to understand that the views of service users are complex, sound and balanced, that they have important things to say about mental health care which providers may not have considered, and that they should have a voice in the organisation and delivery of services.

Our standpoint, our ethics and our attempt to persuade all mean that this report is written in a somewhat polemical style. We hope that our professional audience will be persuaded and that our user audience, whom we have no need to persuade, will enjoy it. In case there are any readers who think our process is an example of very 'soft' research, please turn to Appendix A where more 'hard' issues of method are considered.

This chapter consists of a series of accounts of the experience of UFM written by user group members. The accounts are printed as we received them, without any editing. We believe that they speak for themselves. The names are usually the person's real name but some are aliases. The name printed is the user's choice. The accounts are grouped by project and the details of the projects appear in chapter 5. There are no accounts from Scarborough as the data presented here is part of a longitudinal evaluation that has yet to be completed (see chapter 5).

Kensington & Chelsea and Westminster Health Authority (KCW) Project Phase 1

Hilary Hawking

We were contacted through various work projects and day centres etc. and were assembled in a smart shiny office block in London's City area, spoken to with Peter's American enthusiasm and Diana's quiet, knowing sincerity. We were given a tasty lunch of city sandwiches, fresh fruit and coffee.

Each month we met, became acquainted with each other, all very different people, all with one thing in common: we had been patients in hospital. Sometimes there was friction, a rush to compete with memories fraught with emotion, at other times we joked sharing private but communal anecdotes.

We role-played, practised interviewing, and gradually the questionnaire evolved, was discussed, altered and finally agreed upon. Then we ate sandwiches, fresh fruit and drank coffee.

Interviewing 'proper' began. Could I remember where I was from and why I was asking so many personal questions? Would I be listened to and get answers? Would we both last out?

I entered various establishments – a posh hospital in Roehampton, a lonely, shabby hostel room, shiny hospital units and a depressing social service complex.

I was greeted by staff sometimes with genuine warmth but more often with arm's length indifference, politeness or dubious respect.

Most interviewed were at first cautious, wary of the questions but upon admitting that I too had been a patient and all was confidential, were glad to talk freely, to give accounts of experiences – both good and bad.

They answered, suggesting improvements and changes; also expressing gratitude to those who had been good to them. From some rushed a torrent of feeling, emotion and ideas; others were more reserved, cagey and cautious; but all finished the questionnaire.

The interview over, compensation of £5.00 paid and for most surprise at how enjoyable it had turned out to be; surprised that they might even have a say in their own future; and relief too for unloading a big chunk of their life.

Each month we met, giving accounts of how they went – or not as the case may have been. And some were returned to.

They had been a challenge, sometimes demanding, always fatiguing, sometimes funny or sad often giving rise to my own emotional memories. But I always found them rewarding and worthwhile. And again there was the tasty city sandwiches, fresh fruit and coffee.

Many thanks to the group and especially to Diana and Peter for their insight and encouragement; and let's hope some good will come out of all the time and effort that went into gaining this information.

Esther Rogers

When Dr Diana Rose came to SMART to recruit members to take part in the Sainsbury Centre's survey I was rather unsure about the prospect of interviewing fellow users. I have suffered from a manic depressive illness for many years and was aware of the problems that might arise if the person I was interviewing was high or deluded but I decided to go along to the first training session and meeting at the Sainsbury Centre in Southwark to see what it was all about. As we went on the group of fellow users became more and more committed to each other and the project in a way that I would not have thought possible at the outset.

When the time came for me to do my first interview, Diana Rose came with me as the young man had requested to be interviewed at home. I remember feeling very apprehensive as we made our way there and not at all sure of myself or if I would be able to complete much of the questionnaire. I need not have worried, we stepped into a beautifully kept and furnished flat and the young man, although severely obsessional and deluded in some ways, made us very welcome and made cups of tea. He was delighted to talk about his illness to a fellow user. It was quite an inspiration for us to meet him as with the help of his CPN he was able to run his flat and his life in a way that would not have been thought possible a few years ago.

I was very fortunate as my interviewees – though all quite different – were very nice people. All seemed pleased to talk to a fellow user whom they could easily relate to and share experiences with, and where they were able to relax and speak out. This was particularly the case regarding the embarrassing topic of treatment by the police when ill and most complained of unnecessary force being used and rough treatment. This was particularly sad in the case of three quite slightly built women, two of whom had been held down and handcuffed when there were several officers present to restrain them, if necessary.

Most people were very grateful for the support given by their CPNs and keyworkers though there was confusion about the Care Programme Approach and exactly what it meant, and the roles that different workers played, and who they should approach in a crisis.

I would like to close by relating the case of one man who also impressed me with the way he was coping with his life and his illness. He was full of praise for everyone on his multi-disciplinary team. He had suffered from paranoid schizophrenia for many years – often hearing voices which he thought came from space ships and shutting himself away. But with the help of his psychiatrist and the current medication, he was now able to live a normal life in a flat with the support of his family and ethnic community. He was full of praise for the social service team, because they were always there to help and advise when he needed them.

I found that doing the interviews was a worthwhile and confidence building experience for me and I am so glad that I decided to stay with the team and take part in this.

Pat Kapellar

I had a breakdown nearly four years ago after depression. I made a full recovery with the help I received at the Gordon Hospital – for which I will always be grateful.

I had never interviewed anyone before so, despite the interesting and enjoyable workshops we had at the Sainsbury Centre, I must admit I felt a little apprehensive. I need not have done. I found the work interesting and rewarding. I was surprised at how keen the service users I saw were to help to do something that would improve the mental health service. I did seven interviews, each person being very different – from a young man in his early 20s who wanted desperately to return to a normal life and the chance to work, to a lady in her middle-50s who, through a breakdown, had lost her occupation, having had it for 20-odd years. Her only ambition was to get a flat where she could be happy.

The result of doing the interviews is that I feel confident that this survey will provide valuable information and give the service user a better quality of life.

KCW Project Phase II

Pat Kapellar

I've interviewed a number of service users over the past two and a half years, some of whom were under heavy medication and some who were convinced they had no reason to be in a psychiatric hospital. The latter users almost convinced me!

My own experiences of being a user have made me more aware and I was able to ask questions in a sensitive manner so as not to upset the interviewee.

The service users, on the whole, were anxious to complete the questionnaire, especially when I told them what a tremendous difference it will eventually make to the National Health Service.

When I completed each interview I felt a sense of great satisfaction – especially so when I've returned to a site I've visited, say a year later, and found improvements in the services I've asked questions about.

Robin Hanau

I have concluded work on interviewing service users.

I found all the people I interviewed very helpful, though many were quite isolated. In their social conditions, more could be done to involve them in meaningful daytime conditions.

Most of the people interviewed were not involved with activities, unlike the people including myself doing the interviews. This, to my mind, shows the importance of the user involvement nationally and internationally which the Sainsbury Centre is involved with.

I found the staff I dealt with were quite helpful though not too knowledgeable about the project. I personally found no formal complaints about medication or benefits. The main problem I identified was social isolation – more should be done about this.

Most of the people I interviewed did not have intimate relations with somebody such as a wife or girlfriend, though I think all the people I interviewed were male.

On the whole the project was rewarding for me and I look forward to a continuing relationship with the Sainsbury Centre.

Rosemary McKay

Points for good interviewing of Sainsbury Centre – Phase II

1 *I cannot stress too much that the fundamental success of good interviewing is:*

a) *Good training*

b) *Ongoing questions researched by the team i.e. covering all aspects of mental health care such as key workers and psychiatric doctors and carers and type of medical care received both in and out of hospital.*

c) *The work done by the administrators in contacting key workers, other mental health team members in advance. The location and time and other necessary details finalised before the interview takes place.*

d) *The client or user's welcome to us when we call and his/her readiness to answer quite exhaustive questions which he/she has not thought necessarily important to their treatment.*

It is important that all this is done to make a success of an interview. The users for the most part were given some idea of what was wanted by the interviewer and could relax in the knowledge that there were not going to be any trick questions.

2 *I nevertheless found that some of the users were reticent in their answers at the beginning of the questionnaire because they did not wish to be thought of as complaining. The fact that we, the interviewers, were or had been users did go a long way to making them more forthcoming in their comments. For the most part I interviewed the client safely on his or her own, often in their own accommodation. I would say that for the most part the user was being more than fair in her/his summing up of the services given to them. Medication did alarm them as they knew they were dealing with very strong drugs. Advocacy was a rarity and they could have complained more about hospital conditions. It seems that when mental health is a problem one's aspirations are limited. If nothing else the interview has alerted them to the need for a high standard to be maintained.*

Opendoor Housing Trust Project

Christine Maude

I enjoyed my experiences as an interviewer and I found my work rewarding because the interviewees were so pleased to see someone who not only came to interview them but also to talk to them. Here was someone who also had mental health problems who could listen and understand what they had to say. Many of the interviewees regarded me as a friend and were glad to talk about their lives after the interviews were finished. They appreciated that the work we were doing was going to be worthwhile.

I felt that my work was appreciated not only by the interviewees but also by the staff at the Sainsbury Centre for Mental Health. However, I really need something permanent and I was disappointed that this did not lead to permanent work.

Jean

Being involved in user-focused monitoring has been a very valuable and enjoyable experience. It has shown me that I am not a useless waste of space, rather that I am a capable, articulate person. There were times when I was unable to do an interview, so would have to cancel. I was concerned that I would be seen as unreliable. My fears proved to be groundless, however. Gabriel, you were so understanding of me and my problems that it has helped give me courage to try something new for myself and help me believe I do have a future. For that, many, many thanks.

As for the actual interviews themselves, by and large they went very well. Having two of us at them was useful because it meant I could get feedback as to how I was coming across. Happily most of the people I interviewed had very few complaints about Opendoor. Two things did seem to crop up more than anything else though. One was that people felt they were not listened to, the other was that staff changes make a very great difference to them, sadly not for the better. One comment I heard was that the worker "spent more time on her nails than on me"!

Listening is a skill which can be taught, but is very hard work. One way of improving people's listening skills is to play the 'Shopping Bag' game, you have to listen carefully to list all the items placed in the basket in order. Learning by play is just as effective for adults as for children.

Staff recruitment is a very challenging thing, but constantly having new staff to get used to is traumatic for vulnerable people. One way to help could be to include clients in recruitment of new staff. I attend the Denbigh Centre and there we take part like this. On the day when candidates are to attend the Centre a group of us, who have volunteered to do so, meet up with them and put questions which are of particular concern to us forward. Later on and in a much less formal atmosphere the candidates join all of the members present for tea, thus enabling everyone to meet and have a chat. Subsequently, we put forward our views to staff, who take them into account when inviting someone to join the team. As two of our choices have become members of the staff team and are popular and efficient workers respected by staff and members alike this could be said to be successful.

Added August 2000

User-Focused Monitoring has led to some surprising adventures for me. Since I started on the project for Opendoor, I have had the opportunity to speak to various groups about the benefits of UFM and user involvement. I actually spoke to a group of 500 people earlier this year! Five years ago I'd never have believed that possible.

I am now a passionate exponent of UFM, and of anything which will help others see just what people like me are capable of and of how much difference these things can make to the lives of so many who are often ignored or rejected by society.

I hope you find my comments helpful.

Giles Martin

My involvement as an interviewer on this project has been mainly positive. The structuring of the questionnaire and looking at the questions was an important and valuable process; however I still think there were too many questions some repeating very similar topics and that represented Opendoor's Agenda and had very little to do with users' quality of life.

The training, support and consulting from the Sainsbury Centre and especially Gabriel has been excellent without exception.

The interviews I conducted for Opendoor were all completed without incident or any problems for me and the staff were all helpful.

The information I received from clients varied from service to service, but for the most part was positive about the staff working there. Some people being completely happy, to others feeling that the staff were managing a difficult situation well.

Generally I wasn't surprised by the responses that I got. The homeless people just wanted practical help and more information about their resettlement and for it to happen faster. While the residents of the longer term care hostels were contented, many had the all too common problem of low self-esteem and motivation so expected little. This in my view will always be the most prevalent and difficult to solve problem of the long term mentally ill or dependent.

The day centre I visited seemed to be a happy place with a genuine family atmosphere.

The community support interviewees again were grateful for the contact and practical help they received. Overall it was the contact of a friendly, understanding person that was most important. At the time some workers had changed quite recently so clients missed their old support workers and were reserving judgement on their replacements.

I think continued user involvement is an excellent idea but should only be done in a business like way; where both the management committee and the user delegates agree the aims and implementation of user involvement and their responsibilities into a written contract. Only then would user involvement mean anything to users and their views would be acted upon. Opendoor should be entitled to commitment from these representatives, should be encouraged to train them and probably pay them as well. If there was any sense of 'tokenism' being employed by the management committee of Opendoor then the project will have been wasted.

User representatives if selected and trained properly can be an invaluable link between users and management. Taking comments and ideas direct to management and being the catalyst for positive social and self help initiatives for the users. They would be able to do a lot to encourage, change and truly rehabilitate the lives of many people. This should be part of the user-rep's role, in other words not just there to demand more things for users, but to take an active role in leading and motivating the people they represent, to challenge and motivate their lives.

Huntingdon Project

Daljit Saini

Engaging in my first interview accompanied by John seemed to be the most memorable. We both arrived ahead of time, ready and able and a bit nervous to do the interview. Having John as the second interviewer there helped in carrying out this important and sensitive job. We were basically going into a challenging situation, i.e. a complete stranger, someone with a severe mental health problem, how well would we be welcomed into their home etc? But there was one thing vital we had in common and that was we had gone through the mental health system ourselves, too, just like the person we were interviewing today. We were invited into the house without any tension at all. The interviewee seemed to be in a very bad way, I presume because of his mental health and age. At that point I felt sorry for him but also praised him for taking part in this interview. I also felt that judging by his condition, this interview would take longer and maybe even difficult to complete. But I was proved wrong slightly. He was trying very hard to understand and answer the questions being put to him. I was always encouraged to clarify each question and wait patiently for an answer. His speech was also difficult to understand which meant that I had to listen carefully for his reply. We did eventually complete this interview and I think it was a team effort between the interviewer and the interviewee. I had shared so much with the interviewee regarding his mental health and in a way got to know him as a person in the time we spent together under these circumstances, knowing that after the interview had been completed we could not see each other again.

Andrew Hall

The user-focused monitoring project provided me with a valuable insight into the lives of people with mental illness – how they coped with life in the community and the support they received from the various caring services. I found that the majority of people I interviewed were resilient in the face of adversity coping with difficulties that often come hand in hand with mental illness e.g. loneliness, isolation and the inability to find an outlet for the complexities of feeling and emotion that are therefore compounded.

I have been impressed with the overwhelming amount of caring that goes on but I have also seen the depth of help and empathy that is still needed in the mental health sector – particularly the need for more out-of-hours services and other areas e.g. the need for more formal and informal advocacy and psychotherapy. Very often, life in psychiatric wards has been criticised as demeaning and lacking in imagination – very often patients are treated with drugs with little or no counselling and talking therapy. Often, ward life is characterised by a shortage of activities, a deep boredom and isolation on the ward.

I hope that the research that has been done will acknowledge the good work that is going on and also encourage positive change within a holistic framework of personal development and self-awareness for patients suffering from mental illness.

John J Hunter (Snr) REMD

I personally believe that the whole 'Huntingdon' project could have been a much better success. However, the whole team, including myself, [of] us 'user' interviewers worked hard together from the beginning under the guidance of Jim Green.

Unfortunately we are well into our second year and should by now be developing our improved skills. What will happen in the future? Are we being shelved or filed away? I also believe we are in need of more locality support here in Huntingdon.

The whole team has been an immense success and we have all worked hard together. However, this project is only the tip of the iceberg, we must motivate ourselves, we all believe that priorities exist whether they be in mental health or otherwise.

As regards the general report, it would probably enlighten us all to learn how much is put aside in local government to finance this project, also how much was the Sainsbury Centre sponsorship?

Yet, considering everything we have all worked together, enjoyed our interviews and are looking forward to the future.

Camden Project

Oscar

One of the first impressions of interviewing was that all interviewees were pleased to see me and some thought that it was good research that needed to be done.

The second impression was "loneliness and isolation", when talking to the interviewees and observing the surroundings of the place they lived.

The third impression was that the Flexicare worker was someone they respected and gave them help they really needed.

About the questionnaire, breaking down to the length of the questions – somehow I had to get to the main point of the question and try to explain it in every day language.

Nicky Roberts

I have just completed my fifth and final UFM interview and feel that I have achieved something really worthwhile. I'm glad I got involved in the project, although I've had my doubts – it's not something I could have ever seen myself doing – having little confidence and feeling I had nothing to offer, having sat for years on the other side of things answering questions in hospital ward rounds or from endless medical students.

The group at the UFM meetings were very supportive and friendly, and with their help and the training I received, I was amazed I was able to contribute with my own experiences as a past user of services. I felt very much part of the project.

My first interview was the hardest as I was so nervous, but it got easier as time went on. I was struck by how honest the people I interviewed were. I'd like to say thanks to everyone who agreed to be interviewed and for being so helpful, and to all my colleagues on the project for all their support.

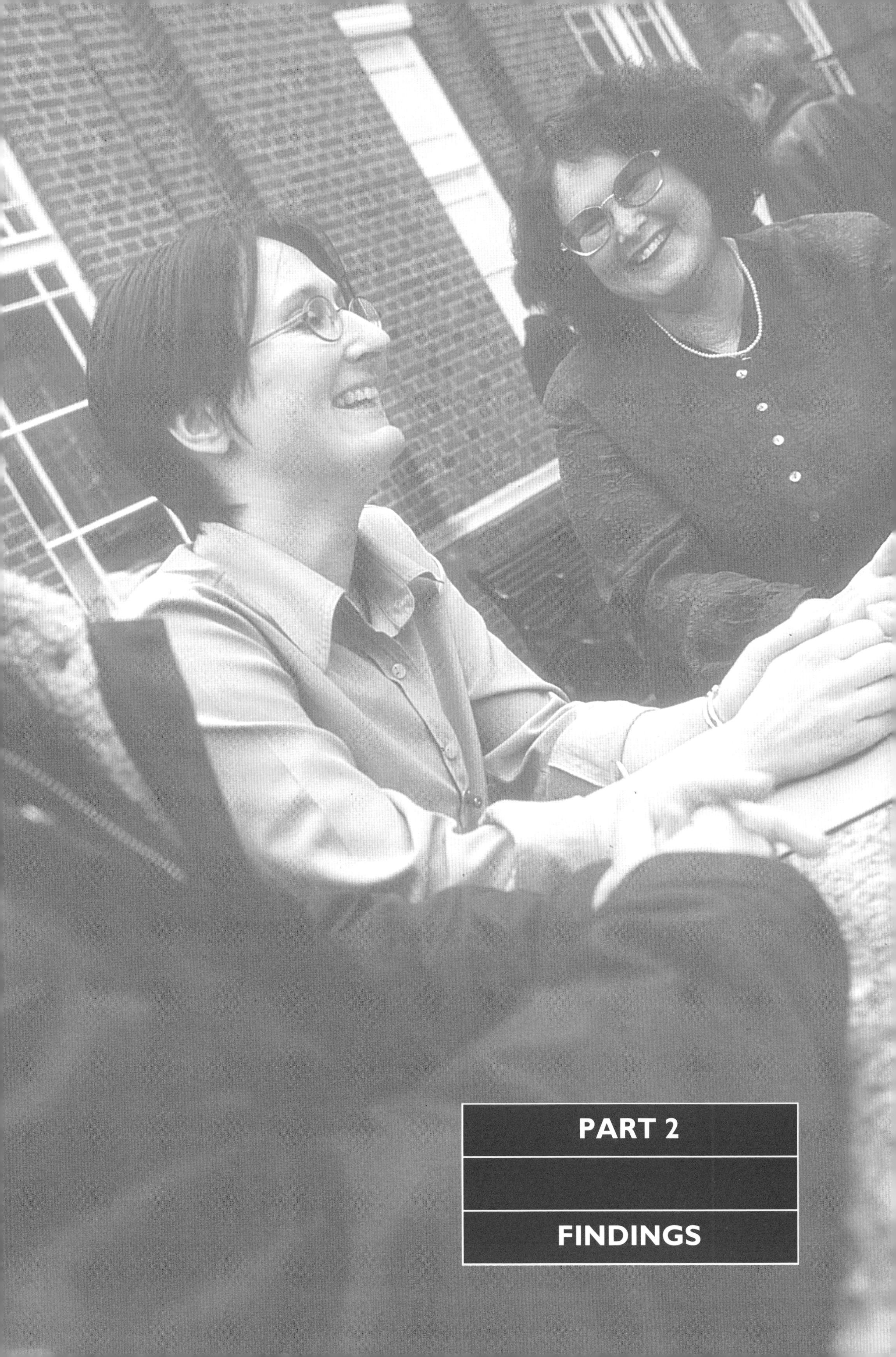

PART 2

FINDINGS

In the following chapters, we present the results of the 'core questions', listed in Appendix C, which were common to six community interview projects. These projects also contained many questions specific to their remit and the results of these were reported to those who commissioned them. In this report, however, we focus on questions which were common to the six sites to try and generate a more general picture. The questions cover:

- information

- the care delivery process

- clinical issues

- mental health crises

- user involvement

- advocacy, health records and complaints

- user satisfaction with care.

The results from the community interviews are quantitative but will be interpreted from the user's perspective as explained in chapter 2. The results from the site visits and the focus group concentrate on the same topics selected from the community interviews and will be presented discursively.

The community questionnaires were all adapted by the local UFM user group to their specific project. Although a set of core questions remains common throughout, there is some missing data where the user group deleted questions because they were not thought relevant to the specific project. This is especially true for the group of Opendoor residential clients for reasons which will be discussed.

In one site UFM has run twice. In between the two applications, we carried out intensive feedback to staff and users of the first set of results. In chapter 13, we look at any changes in responses to questions that might be consequent on this feedback and other policy changes.

We would also like to use our findings to derive a user-focused set of standards to complement those in the National Service Framework. All our core questions can be seen as standards in this way as all the user groups considered them central. We will also try to pick out those questions which seem to have a particular significance for the people we interviewed. To do this we will run statistical tests of association between specific questions and an overall measure of satisfaction with services. This overall measure is a ten-point satisfaction scale with the end-points labelled 'terrible' and 'excellent' which comes at the end of the interview. The questions that made a difference to scores on this scale are discussed in Part 3.

For example, we found that most users said their doctors did not negotiate medication levels with them. However, where doctors did negotiate the users were happier overall with services than those whose doctors simply issued prescriptions. Answers to this question are associated with different overall satisfaction levels. We will argue that the users interviewed, by the pattern of their answers, have shown us that it matters whether doctors negotiate medication levels with their patients. Several other questions also show this pattern of results and we report on these throughout Part 2. The results of the statistical tests appear in Appendix B. A question is identified as of particular importance when a low proportion of users say they receive a particular element of care and the findings show that there is a significant association between this and overall satisfaction on at least two sites.

THE SITES AND THE
GROUPS INTERVIEWED

In this chapter, we describe eight sites where we have carried out UFM projects. They include health authorities, individual trusts, social services departments and a voluntary organisation. We give a description of the site in terms of its geography, economics and social make up. After this, we give information on the characteristics of the group of people whom we interviewed. This includes data on age, gender make up, ethnic composition, length of time using mental health services and the proportion of people having an admission in the twelve months prior to the study. The last two indicators are meant to show how disabling mental health problems are for the group. We did not collect this kind of information for users we talked to during the site visits so the tables refer to the one-to-one interviews only.

The interview asked for a self-definition of ethnicity and it became clear that there was a wide diversity of ethnic groups represented amongst the people interviewed. In the tables that follow we have re-coded this data into a two-way split to show the proportion in each sample who come from a black or minority ethnic community. Of course, this is a gross oversimplification and it overlooks the plurality of ethnicities in contemporary society. However, it has long been argued (e.g. Jamdagni, 1996) that the term black can be used 'politically' to cover all those from ethnic minority communities because these communities all experience ethnic discrimination and that this definition can be used to plan health services. For our purposes, then, our figures indicate those who suffer the double burden of mental distress and racism.

Kensington & Chelsea and Westminster Health Authority (KCW)

KCW was the first of the UFM evaluations and it is the site where we have worked most intensively. KCW is the only site where we have carried out UFM twice: in 1997 and 1999. In between the two evaluations we carried out extensive feedback of our initial findings together with the health authority. We wanted to know if this would make a difference to users' experiences the second time around. So, chapter 13 is devoted to comparing the findings in KCW at the two points in time.

KCW is an inner London Health Authority with a diverse ethnic mix. In KCW we used interpreters for our interviews on four occasions. KCW embraces the extremes of wealth and poverty. For example, it covers the ward where the world-famous store Harrods is situated as well as a ward with one of the highest Jarman scores in the country. The Jarman Index is a measure of social deprivation. There is a correlation between Jarman scores and numbers on the top tier of the CPA in KCW. The higher the deprivation, the more people on the top tier of the CPA. Since our interviewees were selected from the top tier of the CPA, it follows that they tend to come from the more deprived areas in the authority.

In KCW we carried out both one-to-one interviews and site visits. In 1997 we interviewed 59 people and in 1999 we interviewed 77 people. The people were different on the two occasions. All those who were interviewed were on the top tier of the CPA and the total CPA populations were the databases from which we randomly sampled. Tables 1 and 2 show the characteristics of the people who were interviewed.

Table 1 Characteristics of the group of users interviewed in KCW in 1997	
Feature of the group (Total interviewed = 59)	
Average age	43 years
Gender – percent male	64%
Black or minority ethnic group	62%
Average years using mental health services	11 years
Inpatient in last year	63%

Table 2 Characteristics of the group of users interviewed in KCW in 1999	
Feature of the group (Total interviewed = 77)	
Average age	43 years
Gender – percent male	66%
Black or minority ethnic group	57%
Average years using mental health services	10 years
Inpatient in last year	50%

The two KCW samples are very similar and the characteristics reflect those of the total top tier CPA populations. We had access to the population databases and so can say that for demographic characteristics at least our samples are representative.

Our groups reflect the fact that on the top tier of the CPA in KCW black users are over-represented by a factor of five in relation to their numbers in the general population. All the results which we will report for KCW (and Opendoor) therefore apply to black users disproportionately. This will be commented upon in Part 3.

The preponderance of men in the groups may be because, in this age of concern with risk and risk assessments, men are identified as more risky than women and thus more likely to be placed on the top tier of the CPA.

The site visits were to four mental health units containing acute wards and day hospitals. Three of the units also had an intensive care ward. One had a work project. The day hospitals provided occupational therapy to people from the acute wards who were considered well enough to participate. In this sense, the units were integrated and we visited them as a totality one at a time. In 1997 we visited twelve wards and spoke with 76 users. In 1999 we visited fourteen wards and spoke with 98 users.

Opendoor Housing Trust

Opendoor Housing Trust is a voluntary organisation providing housing support at a range of levels to people with mental health problems, substance misuse problems and other people who are vulnerable. It operates in the London Boroughs of Kensington & Chelsea and Southwark and so there is some geographical overlap with KCW. Partly as a consequence of this, the economic and social make-ups of the areas are similar. Southwark is an inner city deprived area.

Opendoor provides both residential accommodation and support for people in their own homes through a community support service (CSS). The residential accommodation includes both hostels and a registered nursing home. Not all Opendoor clients with mental health problems actually identify as such and some avoid psychiatric services. The UFM work respected this.

Opendoor asked the UFM team to investigate tenant and user satisfaction with and participation in its services. Although we investigated many other areas as well, this was the specific remit. As a consequence, there is some missing information from Opendoor balanced by an abundance of information on user involvement.

In the Opendoor project we carried out two sets of interviews, a site visit to Opendoor's Day Centre and a focus group. One set of interviews was with CSS clients and one was with residential clients. Table 3 shows the characteristics of the clients of CSS.

Table 3 Characteristics of the clients of Opendoor CSS interviewed	
Feature of the group (Total interviewed = 26)	
Average age	50 years
Gender – percent male	58%
Black or minority ethnic group	50%
Average years using mental health services	Not asked
Inpatient in last year	36%

The group of clients from the Opendoor CSS services are quite similar to those from KCW in their demographic characteristics although a lower proportion have recently been in hospital.

Tenants of Opendoor's residential services were the ones who tended not to identify as mentally ill. The UFM team was told that this was a very tricky subject for these clients and that the very words 'mental health', for example in the title of our organisation, would put them off. The interview therefore focused on their satisfaction with Opendoor services and questions about mental health services were phrased in terms of their applicability or non-applicability to the user. When it came to asking about their personal characteristics, we only asked about age, gender and ethnicity. We did not ask the mental health questions. The demographic characteristics are shown in table 4.

Table 4 Characteristics of the clients of Opendoor Residential Service interviewed	
Feature of the group (Total interviewed = 33)	
Average age	45 years
Gender – percent male	57%
Black or minority ethnic group	43%

Huntingdon

The local trust in Huntingdon commissioned UFM to carry out an evaluation of their services with people from the top band of the CPA. The Trust serves the relatively affluent town of Huntingdon and its associated rural communities. Some of these are a good distance from Huntingdon. The sample interviewed covered a wide geographic spread and this raised logistical difficulties for the evaluation in terms of travelling for interviewers. It is also a reason why the sample is somewhat smaller than the others are.

There is no visible ethnic minority community in what might be called a 'shire' area. One person identified themselves as Chinese. Huntingdon, then, is very different from the inner-London communities served by KCW and Opendoor. We were interested to see whether users' perceptions of mental health services would be different too and this is addressed in the chapters which follow. Table 5 shows the characteristics of the group interviewed in Huntingdon.

Table 5	Characteristics of the group of top band CPA users interviewed in Huntingdon	
Feature of the group (Total interviewed = 20)		
Average age	45 years	
Gender – percent male	20%	
Black or minority ethnic group	5%	
Average years using mental health services	14 years	
Inpatient in last year	40%	

We have already commented on the different ethnic make-up of this group compared to those in KCW and Opendoor. The other difference is the gender imbalance. Whereas the inner-London sites had a preponderance of men, women dominate the Huntingdon group. We investigated whether this was due to diagnostic differences (a high proportion of people with depression) but it was not. The top CPA band as a whole does not contain this imbalance although there are more women than men. We conclude that this is just a chance feature of the group although one which we will have to bear in mind in what follows.

Scarborough

The UFM project in Scarborough was part of a Sainsbury Centre-wide initiative to evaluate the introduction of primary care managers in GP surgeries in Scarborough. These workers have the job of smoothing the path between primary and secondary care. The evaluation is a longitudinal one with baseline data collected before the primary care managers took up their posts and a two-year follow-up, including UFM, being conducted as we write. Despite the specificity of the project, the UFM remit was to look at the whole range of mental health services in Scarborough from the user's perspective. However, the focus on GPs means that some of our interviewees were not in touch with secondary services and not on CPA. We will divide the sample when necessary.

Scarborough is an English seaside town and much of its economy relies on tourism. Hotel and restaurant staff are not well paid, much of the work is seasonal and some of it is done by workers who come in for the summer only. There are some ethnic restaurants but Scarborough has no appreciable ethnic minority community. However, it has a substantial middle class and retired population.

Another important feature of the town from the user point of view is that the local user group recently made a successful lottery bid and Scarborough Survivors now occupies pleasant premises in the centre of town. Scarborough Survivors have been very helpful to the UFM team by providing a meeting space and helping contact potential interviewers. Table 6 shows the characteristics of the group interviewed in Scarborough.

Table 6 Characteristics of the group of users interviewed in Scarborough	
Feature of the group (Total interviewed = 39)	
Average age	45 years
Gender – percent male	32%
Black or minority ethnic group	3%
Average years using mental health services	9 years
Inpatient in last year	30%

The Scarborough group is more like the Huntingdon group than the inner-London groups. Again, there is a preponderance of women although the imbalance is not as great as Huntingdon.

Whatever the reasons, the differences between the inner-London sites and the more rural sites in the people selected for interview should alert us to the possibility that there will also be differences in how these groups view mental health and associated services. In turn, this may reflect real differences in the services.

Naseberry Court

This project consisted in one site visit to an inpatient unit and a discussion group held with six ex-patients. 26 people were interviewed during the site visit. The UFM work was part of a wider evaluation carried out by the Sainsbury Centre.

Naseberry Court is a NHS acute unit situated in a multi-ethnic area of outer London. It comprises 41 beds arranged on two floors and run as one ward. It was purpose-built to re-provide the services of a large psychiatric hospital that had closed. It had been open for just eighteen months at the time of the visit and concerns had already been expressed about the suitability of the building and the standard of care provided. Prior to the site visit, the unit had been locked but the week before the visit a new manager instituted an open-door policy.

Camden

In the London Borough of Camden, the social services department commissioned the UFM team to evaluate the community support service provided by three voluntary organisations. The usual UFM procedure was followed and 29 users of the community support service were interviewed. However, this project was so specific that the user group drew up a completely new questionnaire in order that the interviews would be appropriate. The results are, on the whole, not comparable to those from the other sites. We will refer to this research where it sheds light on the main findings.

Information is crucial to quality of life. Most basically, if it is not known that something is available, it cannot be used, it cannot be chosen. Good information makes effective choice possible. Questions regarding information are therefore high on the agenda both of our community questionnaires and our site visits.

Living in the community for mental health service users involves negotiating a complex web of agencies and resources in order to obtain an adequate income, decent housing, something to do during the day and a way of spending their leisure time. Most users have to do this while experiencing a severe mental health problem and receiving medication, which can slow them down and dull their mental faculties. It is therefore imperative that they have access to sufficient information to negotiate this difficult life in the community. The community questionnaires, in particular, try to cover the broad range of community living with respect to information. However, in the site visits too, access to information was a priority.

Community interviews

Table 7 shows how many users in each site felt they had sufficient information about a range of issues to do with living in the community.

Table 7	Percent of users in six projects who feel they are getting enough information on a range of information issues					
Information about	Opendoor Residential	Opendoor Community	Huntingdon	Scarborough	KCW I	KCW II
Mental health problem/services	84%	NA	45%	41%	42%	58%
Side effects of medication	53%	NA	50%	53%	42%	69%
Housing	50%	74%	50%	60%	55%	58%
Benefits	71%	60%	70%	80%	73%	75%
Work	NA	41%	73%	30%	56%	56%
Community resources	44%	65%	NA	39%	52%	60%

Two questions were specifically to do with mental health. It can be seen that access to information about one's mental health problem and medication and its side effects hovered around the 50% mark. The exception is Opendoor's residential service where provision of information about mental health services is very high.

Information about the side effects of medication is crucial for mental health service users. It is hard to explain to someone who has never taken these drugs what the side effects are like. In the absence of clear information, many users confuse the side effects of medication with serious physical illness. Oftentimes, users say, "I thought I was dying" so severe are the unwanted effects. It is therefore incumbent on psychiatric staff to be very clear with users about what they can expect in the way of unwanted effects and how they can minimise these. It is clear from the figures in table 7 that this is far from a universal practice. This is particularly important when it is not at all evident how much 'choice' users have about taking these medications (see chapter 8). Some of the Opendoor users explicitly told the interviewers that they did not take what was prescribed because of the side effects.

A range of pressures exist to encourage users to take medication. We find consistently that about one third of our users feel themselves to be over-medicated. They tell us that they feel slowed down and that they sleep sixteen hours a day. In such a climate, the least that users can expect is full and explicit information about the costs as well as the benefits of these medications. This issue is pursued in more detail in chapter 8.

There is more to community living than one's mental health problem and its treatment. Income is important. Our respondents were consistently more satisfied with their information about benefits than with any other information issue we considered. This was true across sites. Some told us that they had advice from a specialist benefits advisor.

Another source of income is work. Competitive employment was beyond the reach of most of our informants, not least because mental health service users are stigmatised in the market place. In the areas where we worked, however, there were a range of employment projects. In Huntingdon, users felt reasonably well informed about these projects. In Opendoor and KCW users felt less well informed which is perhaps surprising as the employment projects, at least in Kensington & Chelsea, are well known amongst community mental health staff. It is unclear why this information is not being passed on. In Scarborough, information provision about employment was considered to be particularly low.

Living in the community may involve making use of community resources, especially for people who identify with specific groups such as ethnic groups or who identify as lesbian, gay or bisexual. Community mental health staff should have a ready supply of information about such resources especially where they can meet needs which cannot be met within the service itself. Our evidence suggests that there is room for considerable improvement in the capacities of mental health staff to supply information about community resources to their clients. Again, this is true for every site with the possible exception of the Opendoor community support service.

As we have said, the interview schedules include a general, ten-point, satisfaction scale with the end points labelled 'excellent' and 'terrible'. In KCW at both points in time and in Scarborough, almost all the information questions were positively associated with this scale. That is, those who said they had sufficient information were more likely to be satisfied with services overall than those who said they did not have sufficient information. This was particularly so for information about one's mental health problem, the side effects of medication and community resources. The full statistical data can be found in Appendix B. In the other sites, the absence of a relationship between information and overall satisfaction was usually due to the small numbers involved, especially once non-respondents were excluded.

This finding of a relationship between access to sufficient information and overall satisfaction with services shows how important good information is to mental health service users. Whilst the statistical tests used do not permit us to establish cause and effect, we can say that information is significantly associated in the lives of people who use mental health services with overall satisfaction with community care services. These findings confirm the arguments we have been making throughout this chapter. They will be taken up again in chapter 15 on standards.

Site visits

Naseberry Court

On first being admitted to the unit, most patients reported feeling bewildered by what was happening to them, and had been given little, if any, information on their stay. There was a lack of information about the unit in general, policies and procedures, the treatment plan, named nurse or consultant, how long a patient could expect to stay in the unit and no information on discharge plans.

Patients detained under a section of the Mental Health Act were often not informed of their rights to advocacy or free legal advice. If patients learned about this type of assistance it tended to be from other patients.

Requests for information about medication, side effects and any choice of treatment were generally said to be ignored by staff. There was also a lack of information advertising community advice and support services such as advocacy, legal advice, CAB, housing or benefits advice, interpreting services or self help groups. Patients told us they were not informed that they had a right to an advocate at ward reviews.

Patients said they needed information about community support services as well as housing and benefits advice before being discharged.

KCW I

Users in the acute wards, intensive care units and day hospitals in KCW told us that there was a lack of information available to them. They were particularly concerned about what to expect from ward rounds and why they were not informed in advance of changes to the drug or dosage of their medication. They would have liked written information leaflets on side effects and someone to help them access that information by going through the leaflet with them. Site visitors saw no such leaflets during their visits. Rights under the Mental Health Act were another area for concern. Many users worried about how they would fill up their time once discharged but there was no information about community groups or work or training projects on the wards. Some users wanted a benefits advisor to come to the wards.

KCW II

The second round of monitoring saw some improvements in the area of provision of information. The site visitors observed information leaflets about the side effects of a range of psychotropic medications on display. However, users, though pleased with this, said they would like help in understanding this information as it is sometimes quite technical. Information leaflets on rights under the Mental Health Act were also available on many units and the address of the Mental Health Act Commission was often prominently displayed.

In some wards, there were posters and leaflets advertising work projects and community groups. These included publicity material for black and minority ethnic community groups and advocacy groups. Some units had set up a Patients' Council and its meetings were advertised. Users on the whole said they were now well informed although mixed feelings were evident about the usefulness of Patients' Councils.

Focus group

Opendoor

Some day centre members told us that they had received clear and concise written information about their service. This was felt to be helpful and better than that from other similar services. However, it was thought that this information was only produced in English and consequently of little use to those that cannot read or understand English.

Users of the residential and community support services had less access to information about their service. They felt that clear written information regarding their service would be useful. On the other hand, many said that staff were good at explaining information to them.

Conclusion

In this chapter, we have considered the provision of information to people who use mental health and associated services. Whilst mental health and associated staff cannot be expected to be experts in all the areas considered in this chapter, they should ensure that they pass on all the information they do have in a way that is accessible and clear. The findings presented here make it plain that this is not happening to the degree that it should. Of course, our findings are not uniform and some groups of users feel that they are better informed than other groups. Nevertheless, we consistently find information provision falling short of what at least half of users would like and this has to be the benchmark – if users do not feel well informed they will be unable to exercise choice and they will be unable to become involved in their care. What is more, our findings show that access to good information is significantly associated with how satisfied users say they are with community care services as a whole.

In our recommendations, we state that medical staff should make sure that users have full information about their mental health problem and the side effects of their medications. Information about side effects is now routinely included in prescriptions obtained from high street pharmacies. This should be extended to hospital pharmacies. In addition, inpatient wards should hold full supplies of leaflets on all the medications used on the ward and staff should help users to access these.

It would be helpful if CMHTs centrally pooled and indexed their information supplies and made sure they were comprehensive and up to date. Sufficient numbers of leaflets should be held so that they are freely available to users who should be helped with the more technical ones. Information should also be available in community languages and on tape. Although this would involve extra work in the short term, it would eventually make information provision more efficient.

In this chapter we focus on care delivery and what users know about it. There is a fine line to be drawn between information, discussed in the last chapter, and knowledge. There are two reasons why we have organised these two chapters as we have. First, this chapter on care delivery is much more specific than the one on information. It is about elements of mental health care such as care planning and keyworking. Secondly, in this chapter we are concerned with services that we know the users are receiving. The question is, do the users themselves know this?

Part of the issue in this chapter is about the extent of a common language between users and professionals. It might appear that this does not matter. It does not matter if you know whether the person who visits you is your keyworker as long as they continue visiting. We take the opposite view. If users are to be empowered in the therapeutic relationship then professionals must not hide behind barriers of terminology or keep systems to themselves. It is important for empowerment that the care delivery process is transparent.

The care delivery process we consider in UFM is the Care Programme Approach or CPA. It was introduced by government in 1991 and policy guidance was issued in 1995 (DoH, 1995) and in 1999 (DoH, 1999a). The later publication recommends that users should be involved in auditing CPA, so this chapter is topical.

CPA is designed to ensure that users in touch with psychiatric services get good quality, consistent care. The CPA has three elements: the appointment of a keyworker, the drawing up of a care plan, and the setting of a date for the next review. In this chapter, we shall find out how much users know about CPA and its key elements.

Not everyone in the Scarborough sample was in touch with secondary services and CPA is only for those who receive secondary services. The Scarborough data is therefore based on those on CPA only.

Community interviews

Less than half the Opendoor residential clients were prepared to have anything to do with psychiatry except when they were sectioned. For this reason, CPA was not pursued in detail with them. Of the fifteen who were in touch with secondary psychiatric services, nine knew they were on CPA. Table 8 gives details of users' awareness of CPA and its elements.

Table 8 Users' awareness of CPA and its elements					
Care Element	Opendoor Community	Huntingdon	Scarborough	KCW I	KCW II
CPA	38%	37%	50%	39%	57%
CPA keyworker	40%	70%	38%	57%	79%
Care plan	*	65%	40%	35%	57%
CPA review	35%	6%	26%	16%	37%

*This question was not asked as the interview discussed Opendoor's own care planning process – see paragraph on 'Focus group'.

All the differences in table 8 between KCW I and II, except the first one, are statistically significant. This will be discussed in detail presently. The discussion which follows refers only to KCW at the first point in time.

Our findings show that the majority of users in all sites do not know what the CPA is for. This major plank of the care delivery process has not been explained to them or, if it has, they do not understand the explanations given. Without understanding CPA, users cannot know that they should be involved in it, can invite an advocate or friend to meetings or use it to raise their own issues with their keyworker and psychiatrist.

With the exception of Huntingdon, the majority of users do not know who their CPA keyworker is. They may, of course, know this person as their CPN, their social worker or their psychiatrist. We would nevertheless argue that it is important for transparency in the care delivery process that they know about the keyworking role and what it involves. That is, that their CPA keyworker is responsible, in consultation with them and with other professionals, for ensuring that the care plan is implemented and that all the relevant people are invited to reviews. CPA keyworking responsibilities are additional to those of a CPN or social worker and the user should be aware of this.

Again with the exception of Huntingdon, users tend not to know that they have a care plan. Very few were able to tell us that they had a written copy of their care plan and this includes the Huntingdon users. Government policy is that users should be involved in drawing up their care plan (DoH, 1999a). But if a user is unaware that they have a care plan in the first place, they cannot be involved in drawing it up. With CPA, the care plan is the practical pivot of care. It is a written document which lays down entitlements and duties. It seems to us almost a dereliction of duty to keep such a document from the user whose life it so directly affects.

Dates for CPA reviews should be made at the previous meeting. The overwhelming majority of our users do not know the date of their next CPA review. We can then presume that they are just expected to turn up at short notice. If that is the case, they cannot influence who attends the meetings whereas government guidance states that they should be able to do this. In particular, they may not have time to organise an advocate or interpreter or the date may be inconvenient for relatives. The very low number of users in all sites who know the date of their next CPA review is simply the most glaring gap in the lack of transparency in the CPA process as a whole.

The experiences of the UFM user groups matched that of the interviewees. That is, when we first presented them with the questionnaires they did not know about CPA and they were angry that it had not been explained to them. We also have the impression from our work that staff think CPA is just a paper exercise which increases their workload with no benefit to care. Given this confusion and indifference, we did not expect the CPA questions to be significantly associated with overall satisfaction. They were not.

Site visits

Naseberry Court

The equivalent of the CPA keyworker role in an acute ward is the named nurse system. Each user should have a primary nurse responsible for their care and a named nurse on each shift. This system was apparently not in place at Naseberry Court. Indeed, there is little to say about the transparency of the care delivery process in this unit because users reported very limited interventions. There was felt to be an emphasis on medication only and a lack of alternative approaches. There were few recreational activities. The overwhelming message from the site visit was of users feeling acutely bored.

The CPA keyworker should, if good practice is being followed, maintain contact with clients who are in hospital. We found no evidence that this was happening.

KCW I

As with Naseberry Court, users in the acute units and day hospitals in KCW were not aware of who was their primary nurse or named nurse. They saw their consultant psychiatrist during ward rounds. Many users saw little point to ward rounds, as they felt unable to have their say and felt intimidated. They did not see ward rounds as contributing to their care and one said he thought the only point of ward rounds was to educate medical students.

There was no evidence of CPA keyworkers visiting their clients whilst they were hospitalised.

KCW II

By the time of the second round of site visits, there was a dramatic increase in the numbers of inpatients who knew who their named nurse was and could explain the named nurse system. Ward rounds were no better liked or understood than on the first set of visits.

Advocates and welfare rights workers were witnessed on the wards during the actual visits. We were, however, unsure, whether CPA keyworkers made a point of visiting.

Focus group

Opendoor

In the focus group, the process of individual care planning in Opendoor was discussed. Clearly, this is just as important for transparency of care for Opendoor clients as the CPA care plan is for CPA clients. Users told us that care plans are talked through by staff. It was felt that this process should be done over three or four sessions and not be rushed. Those who were aware that they had a care plan were generally happy with it. Many of those using the Community Support Service were unsure about whether they had a care plan.

No-one participating in the focus group had a personal copy of their care plan, although one person had been told that they could look at their care plan in their personal file.

Conclusion

In this chapter, we have focused on the transparency of the main process which is used to deliver care to people with a serious mental health problem in the UK. When we consider CPA and its elements, we find that there are few occasions where more than 50% of users know about the system and its elements. If the care delivery process is not transparent, users cannot know what to expect from that process or what choices are open to them. Still less can they be expected to participate in the process.

We can only speculate as to why this situation exists. It must be the case that keyworkers are not explaining to users exactly what the keyworking role is, what users can expect them to do and how they can themselves influence their care. We can only surmise that care plans are being kept in professional files, or, in the case of inpatients, in nursing notes. They are not being copied to or shown to users.

It may be that users do not know about their next CPA review because these are not being arranged as they should. But if they are not, then inevitably the arrangements will be at the convenience of the professionals and not the user who will just be expected to fit in. It may not then be possible for the user to exercise their right to invite an advocate or a friend to the meeting.

As things stand, the whole purpose of CPA will be lost on most users. It will turn into an ossified bureaucracy rather than a system designed to deliver quality, needs-led care. Users and professionals need to develop a common language and here professionals have a duty to take the lead. This is because they are the ones who currently have access to the specialised knowledge and specialised terminology. Of course, it is possible that staff too see CPA as a paper exercise which only increases paperwork and does not contribute to care. This may be why they do not explain it. The problem is that this would be a unilateral decision.

CLINICAL ISSUES

In this chapter, we look at forms of help available from psychiatric services. The issue of medication, which was discussed in the previous chapter on information, dominates this section. This is because nearly all our users were on some form of psychotropic medication and because, as we shall see, there are few alternative treatments available. Clinical issues provide a focus around which UFM and professional research can be compared. Many of the questions dealt with in other chapters are simply ignored in the more orthodox literature. But professional research does address the issue of treatments, especially medication. We hope to show that user-defined questions and user-focused interviews give a picture of psychiatric treatment that is quite different to that which results from professional research. The chapter is divided according to assessment, medication and non-medical forms of treatment.

The Opendoor interview schedules were designed to assess users' perceptions of and satisfaction with the housing and support services provided by the organisation. In addition, many of the residential clients did not identify as psychiatric services users. For these reasons, clinical issues were not pursued in these interviews and, for the most part, there is no data on this area from the Opendoor clients.

Assessment

Since at least the publication of the NHS and Community Care Act, 1990, it has been policy that assessment should be needs-led. However, there is reason to believe that there are obstacles to this. Perkins and Repper (1998) argue that the move to needs-led assessment is simply a semantic sleight of hand. 'Needs', they argue is just a new word for 'problems' and the focus in assessment continues to be on professional definitions of problems which can be squeezed into available services. Perkins and Repper argue that a true needs-led approach would recognise that many needs should be met through ordinary daily living solutions and not mental health services which may be seen as stigmatising. For example, in an earlier report (Rose, 1996) on stigma, one user said that he took two buses to get to his day centre so that his neighbours would not know where he was going.

Beihal, Marsh and Fisher (1992) show how even those social workers committed to a needs-led approach continue to define their clients needs in terms of their own professional categories, believing they know better than their clients what the 'real' needs are. They are also influenced by what they know is available in the way of services in defining needs and problems.

The UFM community interviews ask two questions about assessment. First, simply, whether the user believes their needs have been properly assessed. Secondly, and in an attempt to find out whether the assessment was problem-focused or 'needs'-focused, we asked the users whether their strengths and abilities were taken into account in their assessment. Table 9 shows the results. The first row of the table shows the proportion of users who told us that their needs had not been assessed at all.

Table 9 Users' perceptions of needs assessment					
	Opendoor Community	Huntingdon	Scarborough	KCW I	KCW II
No assessment	4%	10%	28%	9%	10%
Proper assessment	80%	83%	78%	66%	71%
Strengths and abilities	54%	70%	21%	38%	44%

In all sites except Scarborough, those users who told us that their strengths and abilities had been taken into account were more likely to be satisfied with services overall. Usually the results were highly significant. Statistical details may be found in Appendix B. This is discussed further in the chapter on standards.

A consistently high proportion of service users feel that their needs have been fully assessed. However, with the exception of Huntingdon, a much lower proportion feel that their strengths and abilities were paid attention to in the needs assessment. The extent to which this was done relates to overall satisfaction. It is quite likely that, amongst a group of users with disabling conditions, there is some acceptance of professional definitions of needs. If we had not asked the question about strengths and abilities, a question that comes from our user-focused approach, this shortcoming in the needs assessment process in many sites would not have come to light.

Medication

There is a vast literature on psychotropic medication. Much of it is technical and carried out in collaboration with pharmaceutical companies. However, there is also a large literature which discusses and promotes techniques for persuading users to take their drugs (e.g. Kemp *et al.*, 1996). Motivational interviewing and compliance therapy are but two. It is recognised that adverse effects, discussed in chapter 6, are one reason for 'non-compliance'. The new generations of anti-depressants and neuroleptics are therefore promoted as they are said to be better tolerated and less toxic.

This concern with compliance affects the kinds of questions that are put to users in psychiatric research. None of the UFM groups suggested questions to do with compliance. They wanted to know about choice, respect and dignity in taking medication and how distressing users found side effects. In this chapter, then, we will take a close look at users' perspectives on psychiatric medication.

First of all, we established whether or not the interviewee was taking any medication and then we asked whether this was by mouth or injection. We asked the users if their consultant negotiated medication levels with them. After this, the users were asked if they thought the medication helped them. Those who received an injection were asked if it was given with dignity and respect for them. Next, we asked about side effects. The users were asked if they experienced any side effects and then to mark on a five-point scale how distressing these side effects were for them. The figures in the second to last row of Table 10 show the proportion that marked 'very' or 'extremely' distressing on this scale. The final question asked whether the user felt overmedicated at all.

Table 10 Users' experiences with psychotropic medication				
	Huntingdon	Scarborough	KCW I	KCW II
On medication	100%	86%	90%	89%
On injection	35%	40%	36%	34%
Consultant negotiates medication	70%	44%	59%	62%
Medication helps	90%	69%	64%	66%
Injection given with respect	40%	68%	71%	73%
Experiences side effects	85%	59%	63%	63%
Side effect very distressing	30%	11%	24%	22%
Overmedicated	25%	23%	35%	31%

The first thing to say about Table 10 is that users do not show a blanket rejection, or a blanket acceptance, of their medication. In a user-focused interview they discriminate between different questions and show that they balance the costs and the benefits of being on psychotropic medication. The majority report side effects but a far smaller proportion say these are so troublesome as to be extremely distressing. The majority say that the medication helps them but still a significant minority report being overmedicated. A substantial number of people reported both these consequences. The medical profession would be wise to appreciate that users are not 'lacking insight' or being plain stubborn when they refuse or question medication. There are good reasons for users being resistant while at the same time most realise that it can help.

The vast majority of the people interviewed were on medication. For those on tablets, it is literally part of their daily routine. In the KCW II project, those on injections reported more severe side effects. Medication often dominates the lives of psychiatric service users. We shall see in the next section that access to alternative forms of mental health care are very limited for the people we interviewed. It is therefore important that the issue of medication is handled carefully with users. It seems from our results that almost half the consultants do not take the time to negotiate medication with users. Some users told us that their 'consultations' with their consultants were simply about the consultant writing a prescription.

Just under 40% of the users interviewed had their medication by injection. This, of course, means that they were having the traditional neuroleptics with their well-known short-term and long-term consequences. In KCW at both points in time, users from black and ethnic minority groups were more likely to be treated with injections than users who were white. This is consistent with earlier research which shows that black users receive more coercive forms of treatment (Ndegwa, 1998).

When we asked whether the injection was given with dignity and respect for the recipient, a significant minority (a majority in Huntingdon) said that it was not. The very least one can expect with such a drastic intervention, where 'choice' is often doubtful, is that the process of administering the drug should be free of condescension and disrespect. If an injection is administered by a white worker to a black client in a condescending and inhuman way, this must be a palpable form of disempowerment by mainstream mental health services.

Table 10 contains many figures and there were many individual statistically significant relationships. All of these were in the expected direction. Benefit, dignity and respect were associated with greater satisfaction while distressing side effects were associated with less overall satisfaction. However, two variables met our condition of statistical significance in at least two sites. In KCW at both points in time, those who report that their doctor negotiates medication levels with them are happier overall than those who report that he or she does not. Those who feel overmedicated are less happy than those who do not feel overmedicated. We have seen in chapter 6 that information about side effects is also important and in this chapter that being a black user makes a difference to treatment. Statistical details can be found in Appendix B.

Complements and alternatives to medication

Talking therapies

Recently, a major piece of user-led research was published by the Mental Health Foundation (2000a). It uses quite a different methodology from the one pursued by UFM and does not cover the same issues. However, it shows quite clearly that there is a high demand from users of mental health services for talking therapies and, to some extent, complementary therapies. In respect to these issues, the UFM interview schedules are somewhat lacking. For whatever reason, the user groups who constructed the questionnaires did not consider them to be central. We recommend the Mental Health Foundation report to the reader.

Our interview schedules do, however, contain a few questions on talking therapies. The site visit questions include reference to complementary and alternative therapies. Let us begin by considering a question where the users were asked if they had sufficient access to talking forms of help.

Table 11	Access to talking therapies in four sites			
	Huntingdon	Scarborough	KCW I	KCW II
Sufficient access	55%	5%	25%	22%
Insufficient access	33%	44%	54%	46%
No desire	11%	43%	20%	31%

The figures in table 11 vary. Those for Huntingdon can be accounted for by the provision of counselling, clinical psychology and group therapy services in the Trust. Only two Scarborough users said they had sufficient access to talking therapies. It should be remembered that many Scarborough users were looked after by their GP and it seems the consultations did not include much 'talk'. The figures for KCW are steady over time which gives us confidence in the validity of the question.

Half the users feel they have insufficient access to talking forms of treatment. This is a form of therapy which users value but which they feel they are being denied. When asked what was missing from their care, a high number of users said simply "someone to talk to". By this, they did not necessarily mean formal services but rather befriending, companionship and support. In the Camden work, which we have not cited before, 85% of users valued the companionship and emotional support of their community support workers. These were often unqualified staff. The desire for "someone to talk to" in an ordinary way may account for the significant minority of users who have no desire for formal talking therapies.

For the KCW groups, we investigated whether users from black and ethnic minority communities had less access to talking therapies than the rest. There was no difference and this finding does not support that of the Mental Health Foundation which found that black users are often denied talking forms of help. However, our numbers were small.

In Huntingdon, half the users interviewed had a counsellor and 8 of the 20 saw a clinical psychologist. There may have been some overlap in responses to these two questions. All those who saw a clinical psychologist were either satisfied or very satisfied with the services they received. Four of the users interviewed in Huntingdon attended therapy groups. One was dissatisfied, two were satisfied and one was very satisfied.

The Trust in Huntingdon appears to provide a range of talking therapy services. This compares to two users in Scarborough who received counselling. In Huntingdon, the majority of users are satisfied or very satisfied with the service they receive. Let us look at satisfaction amongst those who received talking therapy services in KCW.

Table 12 Satisfaction with talking therapies in KCW		
	KCW I	KCW II
Satisfied	47%	45%
Neutral	37%	40%
Dissatisfied	16%	15%

Table 12 shows that levels of active dissatisfaction with talking therapies are low. On the other hand, a significant number of users are neutral about these services. Satisfaction does not approach the levels found with often unqualified staff in Camden providing befriending and companionship. Neither does it approach the levels of mutual support amongst users which we discuss in chapter 10. It is important to be careful about what is meant by talking therapies. It is a catch-all phrase that means different things to different people. There is good evidence that users want talking forms of treatment but there is less evidence about what *kinds* of talking therapy are desired. There is some evidence in our findings that not all users want, or are completely satisfied with, the kinds of formal talking therapies offered in clinical practice.

When we carried out the first KCW project, we found a positive association between access to talking therapies and overall satisfaction. Perhaps surprisingly, this association has not been repeated on any other site.

Site visits

Naseberry Court

As we have said already, the main, if not the only clinical treatment at Naseberry Court was medication. Users reported feeling overmedicated and sleeping most of the day.

Good nursing involves talking with patients. Users said there was very little interaction between staff and patients and that nurses were most often to be found in the office doing paperwork or talking to each other.

KCW I

There was a heavy reliance on medication on the acute wards and intensive care units and visitors observed people in bed during the day. However, there was a good deal of OT activity in the day hospitals and this was available to inpatients who were allowed off the wards. The OT activities included community meetings, sports, outings and arts and crafts. Two units had a gym although they were often out of use due to lack of staff.

There was nothing to do for those not allowed off the ward, including all those in intensive care units, and these users reported excruciating boredom.

Many staff were felt to be warm and friendly and accessible to patients. The users placed a high value on the staff who treated them with respect and made time to talk to them. In some wards, users had planned and regular sessions with their nurse. At the same time, some staff were felt to spend too much time in the office and a few users said that there were staff who actively avoided talking to patients.

KCW II

The situation in respect of treatments at the time of the second visit to the KCW wards was similar to the first. The exception to this was that one unit had introduced complementary therapies such as massage and reflexology. These were felt to be beneficial by patients who said they made a welcome change to the medication regime.

Conclusion

We have seen in the preceding chapters, and we shall see in the chapters to follow, that there is a whole range of issues that affect the quality of community care services. Psychiatric treatment is but one component of such services. For example, our users consistently placed comprehensive social care higher on their list of priorities than high quality medical care. Decent housing and an adequate income are just as important to psychiatric service users as they are to anyone else.

Nonetheless, those in touch with secondary psychiatric services confront a situation that is different to most others in our society. Not only do psychiatrists have the power to diagnosis and treat they also have the ultimate sanction of compulsory detention. It is well known that this sanction can be used as a threat against those resistant to prescribed treatment. More than one user had been told, "if you won't have this injection, I will have to get the doctor to take you to hospital".

In this context, it is timely to find out what people with severe and enduring mental health problems think of psychiatric services and how they are delivered. In terms of medication, we found here no lack of insight, no blanket reaction on the part of service users. They balanced the costs and benefits of medication. A majority said the medication helped and yet reported side effects. They cope with the adverse effects because of the benefits. However, the medical profession must begin to accept that sometimes side effects represent a good reason for being resistant to drugs. Feeling overmedicated can have devastating consequences for the ability to get on with life and it should not just be assumed that users must 'put up' with this.

The manner in which services are delivered is also important. Respect, choice and dignity are things that users have a right to expect. Doctors who negotiate medication levels with users have more satisfied customers. Nurses and doctors who give injections with respect for the patient should be the norm. We found a significant minority of people receiving depot injections who felt that they were not administered with respect and dignity. This was doubly alarming in the context of the finding that black users were more likely than white users to receive depot medication.

There is good evidence that users desire talking treatments. Our limited questions in the UFM schedules support this claim. However, we have had occasion to question what precisely is meant by talking treatments and to suggest that some users would rather drop the 'treatment' part of the phrase and focus on ordinary befriending and companionship, on 'someone to talk to', including other users, rather than formal psychological therapy.

When a service user experiences a serious mental health crisis, the response of professionals can be admission to hospital. The shortage of hospital beds means that the crisis has to be serious for this to happen. Many suffer because of this. However, the user movement has long argued that hospital admission itself intensifies and prolongs suffering. As long ago as 1989, Camden Mental Health Consortium (GPMH, 1989) described the injustices and deleterious consequences of acute admission. In 1998, the Sainsbury Centre for Mental Health again documented the inadequate care provided by acute units. Many mental health professionals now say privately that they would not like themselves or their relatives to be treated on acute wards as they currently exist.

As a result of pressure like this, there are now some alternatives to hospital admission scattered throughout the UK. Examples include crisis houses such as Drayton Park in London, which is part of the local NHS Trust, and the home treatment team in Birmingham (Sainsbury Centre for Mental Health, 1998b). There are even a few examples of user-controlled crisis services such as Anam Cara in Birmingham. Very recently, the NHS Plan has made it clear that alternatives to hospital are being taken seriously at national policy level. The fact remains that none of our sites included alternatives to hospital admission in times of crisis. A partial exception is Scarborough, which has a telephone help line called CrisisCall.

When mental health crises escalate and there is no appropriate help, it is possible that the police will become involved and use their powers to detain a person under the Mental Health Act 1983. Police responses to people with mental health crises have been an object of great concern to users, as they are perceived to be disrespectful and use excessive physical force. Training of police officers by user groups is now common.

In this chapter, we look at admission to hospital, both voluntary and involuntary as a subject of a section of the Mental Health Act 1983. We also look at users' choices about the kind of help they would like in times of mental health crisis and at users' perceptions of police involvement in mental health crises.

Hospital admission

The data from the site visits gives detailed information about the experience of being in hospital to add to the picture described above. For this reason, this chapter will depart from the usual structure and begin with the site visits.

Site visits

Naseberry Court

Prior to the visit to Naseberry Court, the unit had been locked but an open-door policy was implemented just before we visited. The users appreciated this. It was the only positive thing they had to say. They told us that the only treatment was medication and the day revolved around the drugs rounds. There were few recreational activities and service users reported feeling acutely bored. Although some users were complimentary about the commitment and attitude of individual staff members, many felt there was insufficient interaction between staff and users generally. Nurses were seen to prefer the environment of the office to that of the rooms which the patients used. Users felt uninformed about their treatment, including about the benefits of medication and its side effects, their rights under the Mental Health Act, and about local community facilities. Users were not much involved in planning their care, and felt their views were generally ignored. Provision for the practice of any religion other than Christianity was limited, despite the unit's location in a multi-ethnic and multi-faith area. The food was felt to be of poor quality with a lack of variety, especially for vegetarians or those on special diets.

KCW

We have already pointed to several ways in which the quality of care in the units in KCW improved between our two sets of site visits. Here we will draw out some common themes.

Users reported feeling very bored with nothing happening to fill their time. This was especially so for those not allowed off the ward which included all those in the three intensive care units and most of the detained patients. This was compounded by the situation with escorted leave. It was not uncommon for consultants to allow two hours escorted leave, only for staff to say they did not have the time to accompany users out of the building. This meant that a significant number of the inpatients were cooped up in stuffy buildings for days on end with nothing to do. There was particular frustration at one site in a residential area where there was a large expanse of open space opposite the unit. This belonged to a private school, which would not let the hospital use it during the school holidays.

There were problems around food and refreshments. Most of the kitchens were locked and users felt that this was an unnecessary restriction. Most wards had installed water coolers but when we visited many of these needed refilling and the cups replacing. The food was generally felt to be of poor quality especially in one unit where it was described as "awful".

Individual nurses were well liked and respected especially when they adopted a respectful attitude to users in their turn. However, it was reported that too many nurses spent all their time in the office chatting with each other and doing paperwork. There were instances where users reported night staff sleeping on duty.

The physical environment was often poor and shabby. Users slept in dormitories with thin curtains between the beds that were often torn. Furniture and floors were covered with cigarette burns and needed renewing. Users complained to us that the toilets and bathrooms were not cleaned often enough.

As we have seen, information provision generally improved between the two rounds of visits. In addition advocates were seen at work on two of the intensive care units. In intensive care units, all patients tend to be detained. The presence of advocates is consistent with the increase in the proportion of community patients who told us they had been offered the service of an advocate while detained (see table 15).

Community questionnaires

In the community questionnaires we asked people if they knew whom to contact in times of crisis and whether they had a relapse plan. We also asked about the process of discharge.

Table 13 shows the percentage in each site who knew who to contact in times of crisis and who had a relapse plan.

Table 13 Arrangements in place for times of mental health crises						
	Opendoor Residential	Opendoor Community	Huntingdon	Scarborough	KCW I	KCW II
Crisis contact	70%	55%	40%	70%	51%	78%
Relapse plan	NA	NA	40%	30%	32%	35%

Let us begin with crisis contacts. There is a large, and statistically significant, difference between the two KCW projects. To pre-empt our discussion of the longitudinal evaluation, we can say that the commissioners were so shocked at the initial finding that only half their top tier CPA users knew who to contact in times of crisis that they were determined to do something about it. They evidently succeeded. Yet table 13 shows that this initial lack of knowledge in KCW was not an extraordinary finding. It is similar to that for the Opendoor CSS clients and Huntingdon's figure is even lower.

We saw in chapter 5 that a high proportion of the people we interviewed had hospital admissions in the year prior to the study. Some of the community interviews were carried out in acute units because the selected interviewee was an inpatient at the time. Many of these admissions were under section of the Mental Health Act. Everybody with such a history should know exactly who to contact if they begin to relapse.

But this should only be a beginning. Users and those who support them need to know the details of what to do in the event of a mental health crisis. Relapse plans are now part of government policy which is only good and proper. Overwhelmingly, however, our informants do not have one. Or, bearing in mind the situation discovered in chapter 6, if they do, they do not know about it. That really *would* defeat the object of the exercise.

The interview established whether the interviewee had been in hospital in the previous year and, if so, asked some questions about the discharge process. It is important that users are happy with the discharge process because the period immediately after discharge has been shown to be one of high risk for suicide and relapse (DoH, 1999b).

The numbers admitted in each site were often too small for percentages to be meaningful so we will simply describe the raw data in these instances.

Seven Opendoor community clients had been in hospital in the year prior to the interview. Four thought their discharge had been managed well and two felt involved in it.

Five users from Huntingdon had been admitted in the twelve months prior to the interview. Three thought that their discharge had been managed well and two had been involved in planning their discharge. Table 14 gives the comparable information for Scarborough and KCW.

Table 14 The process of discharge from hospital			
	Scarborough	KCW I	KCW II
Discharge managed well	20%	53%	57%
Involved in planning discharge	27%	45%	52%
Number admitted	11	28	34

Table 14 and the raw figures for Opendoor CSS and Huntingdon show that users' perceptions of the discharge process are far from ideal. It is when discharge is not well managed and does not involve the patient that we can expect tragedies and horror stories.

Mental health service users are the only group in society that can have their liberty taken away without them committing a crime. Compulsory detention under the Mental Act, 1983, is a serious matter. All the talk of consumerism and patient choice evaporates when it comes to involuntary commitment. We therefore asked our users if they had been detained under the Mental Health Act, 1983, in the year prior to the interview and if so, whether they had been given their rights and offered the advice of an advocate.

No one in Huntingdon had experienced detention in the twelve months prior to their interview. Two people in Scarborough had been detained. Both said that they had their rights explained to them and one had been offered the services of an advocate. Table 15 gives the results for KCW.

Table 15 Detention under the Mental Health Act, 1983		
	KCW I	KCW II
Rights explained	70%	75%
Advocate offered	19%	32%
Number	23	28

The figures under 'rights explained' should be 100%. It is a matter of legality that detained patients have their rights explained to them and that staff ensure that they understand their rights. Depriving someone of their liberty and, usually, compelling them to receive treatment, which they do not want, makes it imperative that the limited rights they have should be fully understood. Of course, staff may feel they have explained a patient's rights but, legally speaking, rights have been adequately explained only when people feel they have been explained.

Low proportions of detained patients are being offered the services of an advocate in KCW although the numbers are increasing. This is accepted as good practice and an independent advocate can often put the user's case in an effective way. A very recent study described in a Reuters Press Release and carried out in Australia shows that access to advocates during spells of inpatient treatment can reduce re-admission (details not available at the time of going to press).

Finally, a high proportion of our interviewees in KCW had been detained in the year prior to their interview. We should point out that though the numbers have gone up a little the proportion has fallen. Men in the two KCW samples were more likely to have been sectioned than women and there was no association with ethnicity.

Crises in the community

Crises have to reach a certain severity before they result in admission to hospital. There are very few crisis services in the community which is why, when crises escalate, they result in hospital admission. It is usual for people to be left to cope alone or with the help of friends, often other users. We therefore asked our respondents what kind of help they would like when experiencing a mental health crisis. The users were offered a choice of five types of help: face-to-face contact with a professional, telephone contact with a professional, advice about medication, a non-medical crisis service and GP backup.

Table 16 Help in the community in times of mental health crisis				
Type of help	Huntingdon	Scarborough	KCW I	KCW II
Professional: face-to-face	90%	86%	74%	72%
Professional: telephone	84%	86%	55%	58%
Medication advice	82%	76%	49%	50%
Non-medical crisis service	87%	90%	50%	53%
GP backup	59%	67%	40%	44%

The type of help that stands out as least appreciated by service users is GP backup. Users in Scarborough tend to appreciate GP backup more than other groups and this reflects the fact that some of them only had contact with their GPs. It is still the least preferred type of help in Scarborough. A recent report by the Mental Health Foundation (2000b) shows that 44% of the users who responded to their questionnaires felt that their GP discriminated against them because they had a mental illness.

This is a worrying situation. In theory, GPs provide a service round the clock, 365 days a year. They should therefore be easy to access. There are, of course, issues around cover and locums but someone at least should be available. Yet approximately half the service users we interviewed did not find GP backup an acceptable form of help when they experienced a mental health crisis. Is this because GPs do not provide appropriate care to users in crisis as the Mental Health Foundation report suggests?

Apart from GP backup, users in Huntingdon and Scarborough wanted every form of help! It is difficult to know if this is an endorsement of a very good service they are already receiving or whether their response points to gaps in services, which they would like to see remedied. The absence in the sites of non-medical forms of help, which are endorsed by users on the questionnaire, suggests the latter.

The responses of the KCW users are more circumspect. The preferred form of help is face-to-face contact with a professional. Whilst this suggests that the users find their mental health workers helpful in times of crisis, it also represents a problem for them when crises occur outside working hours.

In Scarborough, there is a telephone help line known as CrisisCall. However, only 30% of those interviewed knew about it.

If users received what they wanted from services in times of crisis, perhaps detention would not be so widespread. However, the reality is that crises in the community do escalate. It is at this stage that the police can become involved and this is the subject of the next section.

Police involvement in mental health crises

Police officers can become involved with mental health service users for a variety of reasons. For example, Rose (1996) shows that when users are victims of crime, police are often reluctant to investigate because they think the user will not make a credible witness should the case come to trial. In this way, police officers and procedures discriminate against service users.

Police also become involved with users when they are experiencing mental health crises in a public place. They have the power to detain for 72 hours in a 'place of safety'. In UFM studies, it is this aspect of police involvement that we investigate. First, we ascertained if the user had contact with the police in the context of their mental health problem. Then we asked if they found the police helpful, whether or not they were treated with dignity and respect and whether unnecessary physical force was employed.

No one in Huntingdon had contact with the police in the context of their mental health problem.

Table 17 Police responses to mental health problems			
	Scarborough	KCW I	KCW II
Helpful	46%	56%	61%
Dignity and respect	50%	68%	70%
Unnecessary force	70%	42%	40%
Number	11	38	50

The first thing to say about table 17 is that an alarmingly high proportion of people in KCW have contact with the police because of their mental health problem. If these two samples are representative of the top tier of the CPA as a whole, and we have reason to think that they are (see Appendix A), then local police are doing a lot of work with mental health service users. In the first KCW sample, a higher proportion of men than women said they had contact with the police because of their mental distress. This finding was not replicated the second time and no sample revealed a relationship with ethnicity. However, in assessing these relationships it has to be borne in mind that black people and men are over-represented in the inner-city samples in the first place.

The majority of the users think they are treated with dignity and respect by police officers but two fifths think that unnecessary physical force was used with them. There were stories of people being handcuffed and put in half-nelsons and bundled into police vehicles. Just over half the KCW users found the police to be helpful overall.

In Scarborough, the numbers are small. Still, nearly three-quarters think unnecessary physical force was used with them and, unlike KCW, only half think they were treated with dignity and respect.

Conclusion

A mental health crisis represents a serious disruption to a user's life. The manner in which crises are responded to can affect their course. A helpful response will limit the crisis whilst an inappropriate response will prolong the distress. Many have argued that the inpatient experience, if not actually prolonging the crisis, is particularly difficult to endure whilst the crisis is running its course. The evidence from our site visits is that the inpatient experience is very problematic, especially for those who are detained. The intervention of the police as a crisis escalates can also make matters worse.

If a crisis results in admission to hospital, the process of discharge then becomes critical. If discharge is not managed well, with good preparation and community links put in place and the user themselves involved, then the situation is ripe for tragedy. The Confidential Inquiry into Homicides and Suicides by Mentally Ill People (DoH,1999b) found that most suicides by people with mental health problems occurred in the week following discharge from hospital, many of them on the very day after discharge. Poorly managed discharge is also responsible for the 'revolving door' syndrome, where users find themselves back in hospital only weeks after discharge.

The arguments for alternatives to hospital admission in times of mental health crisis are now very strong. Crisis houses and 24-hour home treatment teams have been shown to be effective in keeping people out of hospital. The recently published NHS Plan promises access to crisis resolution teams for all users. However, only a few examples have so far been set up and most people do not have access to a service of this kind at present. The users interviewed indicated that they would find such a service helpful, even though they probably did not know very much about what it would entail. User preferences and evidence from alternative services suggests that there is certainly a role for alternatives to inpatient treatment.

But the reality is that inpatient services will remain, especially for those who are detained. In effect, inpatient units may become sink services for the most distressed as others take up places in alternative services. We suggest that users should be involved in training inpatient staff for we do not believe that the majority of these staff are ill motivated. Rather institutional inertia results in less than optimum care. Finally, we suggest that users should be involved in training the police about mental health problems.

User involvement in the planning and delivery of mental health services has been called for since the inception of the UK users' movement. That inception is often seen to be marked by the WHO conference held in Brighton in 1986 (Campbell, 1996). Further consolidation took place at the Common Concerns conference, held in the same town, two years later. Providers as well as users were present at both conferences and sometimes there was intense conflict. Still, speaker after speaker from the user side called for greater empowerment of mental health service users and made it plain that involvement in the planning and delivery of services was crucial to this. International speakers, notably from the Netherlands, told the delegates what had been achieved in their countries and this was an inspiration to the fledgling UK movement. Publications on user empowerment and involvement began to appear (e.g. Read and Wallcraft, 1992) and we have used the ideas contained in such publications in what follows.

Nearly fifteen years after the events in Brighton, patient empowerment is now high on the UK government's agenda. It is at the centre of the new Plan for the NHS (DoH, 2000). In a recent speech, the Secretary of State for Health, Alan Milburn, declared that, "the patient is King". Given the draconian measures proposed in the Green Paper on Reform of the Mental Health Act, and the principles which it contains, it is unclear how far 'kingship' is meant to apply to psychiatric patients. Still, these ideas are not new. The NHS and Community Care Act, 1990, stated that empowerment and involvement of the end-user was to be a priority. The new NHS Plan accordingly puts patients and patients' representatives in positions of influence at all levels of the NHS.

It would seem then that there is a consensus around the importance of user involvement and empowerment. In this chapter, we investigate how this is being implemented on the ground in our seven sites. We begin with an examination of user involvement at the individual level, in the care planning process. We have already seen in chapter 6 that this process is far from transparent to users and this should strike a note of caution when looking at levels of user involvement. Next, we look at involvement in the running of specific services. Here, we take day services and residential services as examples. Do users feel involved in the planning and organising of the day services that they attend or the hostels in which they live? Finally, we look at user forums in the community and how influential users feel them to be. We will take a close look at user involvement in Opendoor specifically, as this was part of the remit of this particular study.

Individual level

Chapter 9 considered involvement in discharge from hospital. Table 18 shows the percentage of users in each site that felt themselves to be involved in the care planning process and the CPA review process. For Opendoor, the care planning process considered is Opendoor's own. For the other sites, it is the CPA care planning process.

Involvement	Opendoor Residential	Opendoor Community	Huntingdon	Scarborough	KCW I	KCW II
Table 18 User involvement in care planning and CPA reviews						
Care plan	39%	30%	47%	21%	22%	23%
CPA review	NA	NA	6%	18%	2%	10%

The figures in Table 18 show a very low level of user involvement when it comes to individual care. Less than one third of the respondents said they were involved in drawing up and reviewing their care plan. We saw in chapter 7 that a majority of users were unaware that they even had a care plan. Since this is the piece of paper around which care is supposed to be organised and implemented, and services are now supposed to be needs-led, it is imperative that users be involved in the care planning process. It would appear that the demands of the user movement, and rather belatedly the demands of policy makers, are falling on deaf ears when it comes to the day-to-day organisation and delivery of services.

The above comments apply even more to the CPA review process. This is an opportunity for users to have an influence on who attends meetings, how their needs are defined and how they are to be met. It is an opportunity for users to ensure that 'needs' is not just another word for 'problems' and that the service they get is led in terms of their definition of their needs and not services definition of their problems. It also is an opportunity to negotiate with service providers over what the user requires and, just as importantly, what they deem inappropriate. The figures in table 18 show a consistent picture of an almost total lack of involvement of people with severe and enduring mental health problems in the CPA review process. Other questions asked in this part of the interview schedule support this picture. Users tended not to know they could bring an advocate to the meeting and they felt the CPA review process rarely covered what they wanted it to cover. Perhaps staff think CPA reviews do not accomplish much and perhaps they don't as currently set up. But users have the right to make their own decision about this and to do so they need information and the opportunity to be involved.

We tested the association between involvement in care planning and overall satisfaction. The results showed that in Opendoor community services, Huntingdon and KCW at both points in time, those who were involved in the care planning process were more likely to be satisfied overall with the services they were receiving. Statistical details can be found in Appendix B.

Our finding of an association between general satisfaction and involvement in the care planning process cannot be used to make statements about cause and effect. Moreover, this was the only involvement measure we were able to assess since, as is clear from the table, the numbers for the other variable are too small. But we can say that involvement at the individual level of service planning and delivery is associated with how happy service users are with community care as a whole. This is important because it belies the view that care planning, if not all of CPA, is a waste of time.

Service level

In this section we look at involvement in the organisation of day services for Huntingon, Scarborough and KCW. For Opendoor residential services, we will look at involvement and the perceived effectiveness of tenants' committees. For Opendoor Community Services, we shall look at the service-specific users' forum organised by Opendoor.

Day services

Since the numbers of users in the different sites who attended day centres varied, and sometimes was very small, we will give raw figures as well as percentages in table 19.

Table 19 User attendance and involvement in day services				
	Huntingdon	Scarborough	KCW I	KCW II
No. attending	11	8	26	35
No. involved	0	2	11	14
% involved	0%	25%	42%	40%

Day services do not suit everyone. We use them here simply as an example of a particular level of organisation of services in which users can become involved. At the same time, even if day services are not everyone's cup of tea, when people are isolated in the community and denied access to the labour market, they provide somewhere to go to and a means of passing the day.

In the four sites considered above, user involvement in the organisation of day services never reaches 50%. Indeed in Huntingdon, not a single user felt involved in the running of the day service. Five users in Huntingdon described the local day service as 'patronising'. In an era when providers are being encouraged to set up user forums in their services and involve users in everything from the organisation of activities to the appointment of new staff, we find from our respondents a perception that services are something that is 'done to' them, rather than with them. Lack of involvement at the individual level is here mirrored by lack of involvement at the service level.

Opendoor tenants' meetings

The residents in Opendoor housing were asked some questions about the tenants' meetings in their houses. Thirteen of them, or 39%, said they were unaware of such meetings. We are not sure if this is because the meetings were temporarily suspended in some houses or because they were badly publicised, especially to new residents. Whatever the reason, this figure suggests a lack of clear information which is a precursor to involvement.

The residents were asked how influential the meetings were for the running of the houses and hostels. Nine people, or 27% of those who knew about the meetings, thought they had no influence at all. A further 9 people thought that the meetings were mildly influential. Two users thought that they were very influential.

Opendoor user forum

Opendoor organises a users' forum for its clients and the Opendoor CSS interview asked respondents about this forum. They were asked if they knew about it and, if so, how influential they thought it was. Twelve people, or just under half the group, knew about the users' forum. This again suggests an absence of clear information.

Most people said they did not know how influential the forum was, eight responding in this way. Two said they thought it was influential, one mentioning repairs, and two thought it was not.

Community level

The interview schedule asks informants if they know about their local user involvement group and how influential they think it is. Clearly, responses to this question will depend on how well developed local user forums are. For instance, Scarborough Survivors has a large building near the centre of the city whilst in the Westminster section of KCW the user involvement groups have closed memberships.

Table 20 shows the percent of each group who were aware of their local user forum and the percent who believed it to be influential in the organisation and delivery of services.

Table 20 User involvement groups and their influence				
	Huntingdon	Scarborough	KCW I	KCW II
Aware	20%	68%	55%	58%
Influential	7%	5%	11%	6%

In Huntingdon, the user group is not well known. This may be because it is a rural site and both publicity and attending meetings can be difficult. In Scarborough, two thirds of users know about Scarborough Survivors. This is a well-funded group with prominently placed premises. In KCW, at both points in time, just over half the users are aware of local user forums. This is a higher proportion than we would have expected because two of the major user groups in KCW have closed memberships and are not well-publicised.

It is very plain from table 20, however, that individual users do not believe that these groups have an influence. It is perhaps surprising that this is so for Scarborough as Scarborough Survivors has the resources to get the voice of local users heard.

It is well known that local user involvement groups face a constant struggle for existence. They are not well-funded and funding is usually short term. They usually do not have premises and equipment. This can lead to a few very committed individuals doing the bulk of the work. Often, these individuals face the added burden of being called 'unrepresentative' by planners and providers. This becomes one reason for not listening to what they have to say.

Individuals who take on this work have to learn fast and sometimes they can become 'professionalised'. This can lead to the group and its leaders becoming remote from its constituency. In fact, the most common response to our question on the influence of user groups was 'don't know'. Ordinary service users simply do not know how influential their local user involvement groups are. Publicity and information are important for feeding back successes as well as pointing to areas where planners and providers are stonewalling. But groups need support to do this otherwise consultation and involvement will remain as token as it has been for other client groups (Barnes, 1997).

Users do not only come together to influence planners and providers. The user movement has a long tradition of self-help and those involved in user forums often attend for social, rather than political, reasons. Group meetings can provide an opportunity for users to come together and discuss issues of common concern. And, of course, users come together in sites in the community outside formal forums. We therefore asked our respondents if they found other users supportive and helpful. Table 21 shows the results. The question was not asked in the Opendoor interviews, which had more specific questions about fellow residents.

Table 21 Percent of users in four sites who find other users supportive and helpful

	Huntingdon	Scarborough	KCW I	KCW II
% affirmative	90%	90%	71%	67%

The figures in table 21 provide a strong endorsement of the value of self-help and mutual assistance. The proportion endorsing the help of other users is, on the whole, higher than of the satisfaction ratings given to mental health professionals and explored in chapter 12. The exception to this is community support workers in Camden. Users may be unclear about the value of user involvement groups in the planning process but they are very clear about the support and encouragement that they receive from their fellow users.

Organisation level

Opendoor – focus group

A few people in the focus group knew that if they needed to they could contact a project manager or someone at head office. Many felt that a help-line or single point of contact for Opendoor services would be a good idea. It was felt that input into changing practice and future development of the organisation could possibly happen during community meetings.

Few people knew about the Board of Management. Many felt that user representation on the Board was a good idea, but for that person(s) to be representative it would be helpful if they had visited the different services and met people to find out what issues need raising.

No service users were aware of the organisation providing training or support to increase user participation in the running of Opendoor.

Only one person in the focus group knew the name of the Director of Opendoor. She commented that he had visited the Day Centre recently, which was welcomed.

Site visits

Naseberry Court

There was no evidence of any user involvement in care planning or treatment at Naseberry Court. Naseberry Court did not have a Patient's Council, although the review team recommended that one be set up.

KCW I

As we have already said, users in KCW did not feel able to participate in ward rounds. No user told us that they were involved in the care planning process. Those who had access to the day hospitals reported that there were community meetings where activities were planned, for instance, outings.

At the time of the first site visit, one of the units had an active Patient's Council.

KCW II

Ward rounds continued to be an issue for users in KCW. Care planning fares little better with many users unaware that they had a care plan, let alone feeling involved in it. However, at the time of the second visits, users in one unit in particular reported access to alternative and complementary therapies which had been introduced as a result of pressure by a local user group.

At the time of the second visits, three of the four units had developed Patient's Councils. Users expressed mixed feelings over how much influence these Councils had. It was felt that staff confined their influence to trivial matters and not those users saw as important, for example, access to the kitchen at all times. Attending Patients' Council meetings was difficult for those confined to wards and intensive care units. It was felt that staff did not make a priority of escorting these patients to meetings.

Conclusion

This chapter opened by suggesting that a consensus now exists on the importance of user involvement at all levels of mental health care. Our findings in our seven sites, on the other hand, show that involvement is extremely low. Whether it be at the level of individual care planning, at the level of services such as day services or residential services, at the level of whole organisations such as a voluntary sector charity or a mental hospital or even at the level of the planning and delivery of community care itself, users do not feel involved in their care. What is more, our findings are consistent over seven sites as varied as whole communities, housing organisations and acute units.

Is user involvement just a paper exercise? This is exactly what care planning appears to be. And yet the small numbers of people who were involved in planning their care were significantly happier overall with services than the large majority who were not. A paper exercise is certainly not what the UK user movement intended when it first made its demands. It is not what local user groups intend today as they meet with planners and providers. It is not even what the government intends as it 'puts the patient first'.

We need to think seriously about how greater involvement and empowerment can be brought about. Both information and transparency in the care delivery process are important prerequisites for making empowerment possible. We have seen that they are not yet fully in place. Involvement and empowerment also involve changes to the client/helper relationship so that users are able to have an influence in defining their own needs and suggesting solutions to these needs (which may not be mental health services). Equally, planners need to make sure that they are avoiding tokenism and that user representatives have sufficient training to handle complex meetings and sufficient resources to feed back to their constituencies. Such changes in relationships involve handing some power back to the users but they also promise greater partnership in mental health services. Guidelines for joint working between users and purchasers and providers are included in a recent report by the Sainsbury Centre for Mental Health (2000).

We have made much in this chapter about the role of the UK (and international) user movement in pressing for greater involvement and empowerment. But we should not be afraid to point out that the user movement remains in a fragile situation. Approximately half our informants knew about their local user groups but they were unclear about how much influence they had. This is a two-sided problem. On the one hand, authorities, including government, need to make resources available so that user groups can receive the training and support necessary to be effective in the process of influencing services. Much of what happens at the moment remains at the level of tokenism. At the same time, user groups need resources to communicate with their members and wider constituencies. However, user groups themselves also need to make this happen. There can be a tendency to become so focused upon the demands of planners and providers that the wider constituency is forgotten. Local users should not, as we have found, be ignorant about the activities of their local groups.

Not everyone wants to be politically active. In this, mental health service users are no different to all other sections of the population. But users share a common history and a common experience of services. They also share the experience of being stigmatised and socially excluded (Rose, 1996). Like many in this position, mental health service users can gain encouragement and support from sharing these experiences with each other. We found in our results that the vast majority do exactly that. Self-help can be just as important for psychiatric service users as involvement in running services or influencing decision makers.

Finally, it can be pointed out that some groups have become disenchanted and given up trying to be 'involved' with services. They have decided to stand outside them and mount a direct challenge in the form of direct action. An example is Reclaim Bedlam, which picketed the Bethlem Royal Hospital's celebration of its long history recently and constructed an alternative, patients' history in the name of the reality of Bedlam.

ADVOCACY, HEALTH RECORDS

AND COMPLAINTS

In the view of the UFM user groups, the issues of advocacy, access to health records and complaints procedures have a natural affinity because they are another route, besides user involvement, to greater user empowerment. However, they have different legal statuses and policy frameworks.

There is no right to advocacy in mental health except in the case of legal representation at Appeals Tribunals for which legal aid is available. On the other hand, the National Health Service Executive Mental Health Task Force has given a weak endorsement of advocacy in mental health through the publication of the Advocacy Code of Practice.

The situation with access to health records is different because this right has been enacted in the Access to Health Records Act (DoH, 1990b). However, this legislation includes a 'harm' condition under which a doctor can refuse access to notes if he or she believes it would harm the patient.

The legal and policy context for complaints procedures is complex and beyond the scope of this report. There is a hierarchy of people to whom complaints can be made and ultimately legal representatives can become involved or community health councils can take on a case. To some degree, complaints procedures may vary according to local circumstances.

If the provisions in the new NHS Plan are implemented, existing measures will be strengthened and some of what is currently guidance will become law. The NHS Plan introduces electronic access to health records (provided the technology exists) and provides for letters between doctors to be automatically copied to the patient. The introduction of Patient Advocacy and Liaison Services (PALS) is supposed to strengthen complaints procedures in favour of the patient. PALS will mean an advocacy service in every Trust but in learning disabilities and mental health this is not to replace existing or future independent advocacy schemes. The details of the relations between the two types of advocacy have yet to be worked out.

In light of these ongoing policy changes and especially the very recent nature of the NHS Plan, the data presented in this chapter should be seen as a snapshot in an evolving process. If the Plan does indeed make a difference, these results will not be repeated in the future. Indeed, it is very likely that UFM will be asking different questions.

Findings

The UFM community questionnaires asked about advocacy, health records and complaints. The Opendoor questions focused these issues in terms of the organisation. Users were asked if they knew about these provisions, had made use of them and how satisfied they were with the outcome. Table 22 shows what proportion of users in each site know what an advocate is, knew that they could see (or try to see) the records kept about them and would like to be able to make a complaint if necessary.

Table 22 User awareness of advocacy, the right to see health records and their ability to complain in six sites						
Know about / would like	Opendoor Residential	Opendoor Community	Huntingdon	Scarborough	KCW I	KCW II
Advocacy	46%	46%	70%	77%	42%	59%
Records	Not asked	19%	55%	28%	44%	37%
Complaints	42%	46%	50%	56%	57%	73%

Table 22 shows that about half the users in Opendoor and KCW knew what an advocate was and approximately three-quarters did so in Huntingdon and Scarborough. Lower proportions of users knew that they had the right to access their health records in all sites. The proportion that felt able to complain was constant at around 50%, except for KCW II where it is much higher.

Although the figures in table 22 are not high, a substantial proportion of users in all sites know about the provisions. Those who do not often did not fully understand the question and the terminology used by the interviewer. There is yet again an issue here about information and publicity and this will have to be addressed by Trusts when they introduce PALS and other measures designed to increase user choice and empowerment.

For the most part, only a tiny minority actually *accessed* advocates, their health records or complaints procedures. For instance, 70% of Huntingdon users knew what an advocate was but only 25% had used such a service. In Opendoor CSS, 46% of users would like to make a complaint if necessary, but only two people had actually done so. Because of the very small numbers of people we interviewed who actually accessed these provisions, and are therefore able to say how satisfied they are with them, percentages are meaningless. In what follows we shall present raw data for the most part.

Advocacy

The users who had made use of an advocacy service in all sites tended to split evenly between being actively satisfied, neutral and actively dissatisfied. This may come as a surprise to those who believe that advocacy is unequivocally a 'good thing'. The fact is that 'advocacy' as a term and as a process does not have a uniform meaning. Some users told us that their keyworker or social worker was their advocate and this is entirely different to the kind of independent advocacy which groups like the United Kingdom Advocacy Network promotes. It is highly likely that this lack of uniformity is reflected in the services used by our interviewees and so it is difficult to be very clear about what the data means.

Different models of advocacy in mental health have never been systematically evaluated, still less evaluated from the perspective of what their users want from them. This is a glaring gap in an increasingly 'evidence-based' NHS. We recommend that such an evaluation be undertaken.

Health records

The proportion of interviewees who knew they could access their health records in all sites was low. The total number of users who had actually seen their health records across all community samples was two. However, in those sites where we asked the question "have you ever wanted to see your health records?" 30% answered in the affirmative. (This question was not always asked). It can be inferred that some users do want to access their health records but that, for whatever reason, this does not happen.

When the Access to Health Records Act (1990) was introduced, psychiatric patients were often invoked as an example of the type of patient who would be 'harmed' by seeing them. This can be a reason for refusal of access. Another reason is breaking the confidentiality of a third party such as a relative. Indeed, in the run up to the Act, the Royal College of Psychiatrists argued that psychiatric patients should be exempt from its provisions altogether. If, and when, automatic and electronic access is introduced, is this 'harm' going to be widespread or will it be used again as a reason to make psychiatric patients a special case when it comes to automatic access to notes?

What is the nature of this 'harm'? Jha et al. (1998) found that psychiatric patients were more likely than those with a physical illness to say that their notes had the wrong emphasis and to be upset by reading them. They cite earlier work, which showed that patients found psychiatric notes to be 'offensive'. Terms like 'paranoid', 'chaotic lifestyle', 'apathetic and demotivated', and 'risk of violence' are not value-free and they have common sense as well as professional meanings. The question is how far the professional categories are imbued with common sense values.

UFM, as well as an increasing amount of other work, values service users. Adopting the user's perspective and a strengths and recovery model of mental distress will change language. Perhaps then it will not be so 'harmful' for users to see their notes. Indeed, automatic patient access to notes may encourage medical practitioners to think about the language they use in talking and writing about mental health service users.

Complaints

Although table 22 shows that about half the users wanted to make a complaint if necessary (73% in KCW II), only a handful had actually made a formal complaint in most sites. The exceptions were both KCW projects which both had larger samples absolutely and where a higher proportion had actually made a complaint. Even in KCW, however, more people wanted to make a complaint than had actually made one.

There are two distinct possible reasons for this finding. On the one hand, users may want to make a complaint should the occasion arise but so far everything has been satisfactory. They do not complain because they have no reason to. On the other hand, users may want to complain but feel unable to do so. They may fear repercussions such as loss of a service. They may feel that their complaint will not be taken seriously and that they will be branded a trouble-maker. Or they may be simply cynical about the whole procedure and feel it is not worth the effort.

The data allows some teasing out of these issues. The Opendoor users were asked the question "Would you fear repercussions, such as a loss of the service, if you were to complain?" Exactly half answered this question in the affirmative. The other half said they could not imagine ever needing to make a complaint because they were so happy with the service. So it seems that there are at least two distinct reasons for not making a complaint.

The situation with KCW is different. A substantial minority told the interviewers that they had actually made a complaint. Overwhelmingly (81% the first time and 82% the second time) they said the situation had not been resolved to their satisfaction.

The second KCW project turned up a very curious finding. It is impossible to say whether this finding can be generalised because elsewhere the numbers were too small to run the statistical tests. Basically, those who were knowledgeable about access to health records and about complaints procedures were *less happy* overall than those who did not know about these measures. Here is a case where information is related not positively but negatively to satisfaction.

One unexpected finding does not mean much. It could be due to chance. But to find the same result on two related variables is interesting. The experience of the interviewers suggests that people who are aware of these provisions are also very cynical about them making any difference to services.

Site visits

Naseberry Court

There were no advocates available at Naseberry Court and no Patients' Council. Users told the visitors that they felt unable to complain even though there was plenty to complain about.

KCW

In between the two sets of site visits in KCW, an advocacy project was set up. This led to the introduction of Patients' Councils in two units and a third already had one. Users had mixed feelings about the efficacy of these Councils, some telling us that their power was restricted to fairly superficial issues. Users who were not allowed off the ward without an escort were rarely escorted to the meetings.

Advocates were seen at work on two of the intensive care units as we actually carried out our visits.

As we saw in chapter 7, we asked our community interviewees who had had an admission in the previous year whether they had been offered the services of an advocate. The proportion who had been offered such a service increased between the two rounds of interviewing and although the difference did not reach statistical significance, we assume this too is because of the introduction of the advocacy project.

Conclusion

The development of independent advocacy projects has been going on apace as we have carried out these UFM projects. This development has had an effect on some of our findings. Together with the new structures and processes promised in the NHS Plan, this may mean that our findings will very soon be dated. But some caution is necessary. We have seen in this chapter how the 'harm' condition in relation to access to health records is often used to deny psychiatric patients access to their notes or to give them only partial access. In effect, this made psychiatric patients a 'special case' in relation to specific legislation. It would not be difficult for this to happen with the new measures, even if it was only by default. For instance, in a recent study (Rose, Warner and Ford, submitted) we showed how staff in acute and secure provision dealt with complaints of racial harassment by black and minority ethnic detained patients by putting the complaint down to 'paranoia' or 'delusions'. In this way they dismissed the complaint. Presumably this does not just happen with complaints of racial harassment. Getting help from a PALS in an accident and emergency department may also involve labelling for psychiatric patients, for instance those who self-harm may be dismissed as 'attention seeking' and 'manipulative'.

Advocacy, access to health records and using complaints procedures can intersect. An advocate can help with access to notes and with complaints. For that matter, a complaint can be brought against an advocate. It is to be hoped that the measures introduced in the NHS Plan will bring some coherence to these avenues for greater choice and empowerment for mental health service users and that these users will have as much access to the new structures and processes as everybody else.

This chapter is the one that relates most directly to the methodological literature reviewed in Appendix A. Of course, many factors contribute to satisfaction with community care services and we have tried to identify these throughout this report.

We will begin this chapter by examining satisfaction ratings for a range of mental health professionals in the four community sites. The professionals are keyworkers, consultants, junior doctors, CPNs and social workers. Following this, we shall consider community support workers in the four sites, Opendoor CSS and Camden. Opendoor residential clients were not asked general satisfaction questions about particular groups of staff although they were asked many specific questions about staff which are not included in this report.

As stated often in this report, the interview schedules ended with a ten point global satisfaction rating. We will give the average satisfaction rating for each site, bearing in mind that many consumer satisfaction studies in mental health result in ratings as high as 90% and that this 'halo effect' has been argued to be unrealistically high (Stallard, 1996).

Keyworkers

Table 23 Satisfaction ratings for keyworkers in four sites

	Huntingdon	Scarborough	KCW I	KCW II
Satisfied	70%	69%	19%	16%
Neutral	30%	00%	72%	77%
Dissatisfied	00%	30%	9%	7%
Number	14	13	47	62

Table 23 does not show a consistent picture. There is a clear division in the results between the inner-city health authority of KCW and the more rural or small town sites. In the inner city, users are overwhelmingly neutral about their keyworkers. This is not a chance finding. It persists across time. In Huntingdon and Scarborough, on the other hand, users are satisfied with their keyworkers. It should be pointed out that the actual numbers with a keyworker are rather low in these sites.

Consultant psychiatrists

Table 24 Satisfaction with consultant psychiatrists				
	Huntingdon	Scarborough	KCW I	KCW II
Satisfied	55%	77%	22%	21%
Neutral	25%	17%	58%	62%
Dissatisfied	10%	6%	20%	17%
Number	18	18	45	61

Again there is a division between more deprived and more affluent areas. Consistently in KCW, there is neutrality about consultant psychiatrists with equal, and small, proportions being satisfied and dissatisfied. In Scarborough in particular, there is a high level of satisfaction with consultant psychiatrists amongst users.

Junior doctors

In Scarborough and Huntingdon, very small numbers of people saw junior doctors. In KCW, the pattern of satisfaction/dissatisfaction was similar to that for consultants. The main complaint against junior doctors was that they changed so often and appeared not to have read the user's notes.

CPNs

Table 25 Satisfaction with CPNs				
	Huntingdon	Scarborough	KCW I	KCW II
Satisfied	64%	72%	73%	73%
Neutral	29%	17%	22%	23%
Dissatisfied	00%	11%	5%	4%
Number	14	18	37	44

CPNs are popular with the users interviewed. In KCW they are much more popular than medical staff. Again we find in KCW consistency across time which gives confidence in the satisfaction ratings. It is curious that CPNs should be so much more popular than keyworkers in KCW since some CPNs will also be keyworkers. It has been seen that this distinction is not always clear to users.

Social workers

In Scarborough and Huntingdon there were too few people with a social worker to make percentages meaningful. In Scarborough, five users had a social worker, four were satisfied and one was neutral. In Huntingdon, there were seven users with a social worker. Four were satisfied, one was neutral and two were dissatisfied. Table 26 gives the information for KCW.

Table 26 Satisfaction with social workers in KCW		
	KCW I	KCW II
Satisfied	56%	60%
Neutral	21%	23%
Dissatisfied	23%	17%
Number	39	52

In KCW, social workers are not as popular as CPNs but they receive higher satisfaction ratings than medical staff. Overall, there is evidence in the findings about satisfaction with professionals that users appreciate the work of frontline staff.

Community support workers

The numbers of people receiving the service of a community support worker were low and percentages would not be meaningful.

No-one in Huntingdon had a community support worker. Of the nine users in Scarborough who had a community support worker, six were satisfied and three were neutral. Fourteen people in the KCW I project had a community support worker. One was dissatisfied, two were neutral and 11 were satisfied. In the KCW II project, 18 users had a community support worker. One was dissatisfied, three were neutral and 14 were satisfied.

It can be seen that, in the four community sites, community support services were less available to users than professional services. However, it is also clear that those users who did have a community support worker appreciated the service. This finding is consistent with the Camden study, which looked specifically at users' perceptions of and satisfaction with community support workers. Of the 29 users interviewed in Camden, no-one was actively dissatisfied with the service they received.

Community support workers provided support to the Opendoor CSS clients so that they could live in their own homes. These workers received some training from Opendoor. Eighty per cent of the clients said their worker was 'very helpful'. Only one person said their worker was 'not helpful at all'.

Overall satisfaction

Before going on to discuss these findings, we shall consider the overall ten-point satisfaction scale filled in by all users at the end of their interview. Table 27 gives the mean score for each group on the ten-point scale. The mid-point, representing neutral satisfaction, would be five.

Table 27 Mean satisfaction ratings in six sites					
Opendoor Residential	Opendoor Community	Huntingdon	Scarborough	KCW I	KCW II
5.3	7.7	7.0	6.3	6.0	6.3

The first interesting feature of table 27 is that there is no evidence of the so-called 'halo effect'. The 'halo effect' is the term given to findings of uni-dimensional satisfaction questionnaires. These typically show consumer satisfaction with mental health services running at up to 90%. Commentators have suggested that these findings are misleading and do not accurately reflect the user experience. It has been argued that features of the questionnaires and the contexts of their administration account for the high satisfaction ratings.

Our users typically rate their satisfaction on the positive side of neutral. We would therefore argue that UFM as a method elicits more realistic and accurate responses than orthodox instruments. And these responses make it plain that there is much room for improvement in mental health services.

The second interesting feature of table 27 is the consistency of the responses. In this chapter, when we looked at satisfaction with mental health professionals, we found some variation between sites. The overall satisfaction ratings are, however, remarkably consistent. We shall suggest some reasons for this in Part 3.

We have also found throughout this report that overall satisfaction is correlated with a number of other questions. We will argue later that this can tell us something about the features of a good community care service.

Conclusion

It may be that satisfaction with mental health professionals is not always a sensitive measure of how users feel about the mental health services they receive. We have presented the results as if they were satisfaction ratings of different professional *groups*. But the questions were phrased in terms of *individuals* – e.g. 'how satisfied are you with your consultant psychiatrist'. To some extent at least, the answers must reflect the personal qualities of the individual member of staff concerned. In the case of consultant psychiatrists, this could affect overall ratings in small communities as there will only be one or two of them and users' perceptions will be coloured by their personal characteristics. One helpful individual will have a disproportionate effect on satisfaction ratings. This could account for the variation in responses between sites in terms of medical staff.

CPNs, social workers and, especially, community support workers get to know their clients quite well. Relationships are part of the service and so it is perfectly appropriate to ask users about their satisfaction with these relationships. Our results show that, on the whole, frontline staff are appreciated. But these relationships are not the whole of the service. It does not matter how much you like your CPN, if you cannot get out of bed because of being too sedated this will affect how you see services as a whole. It will certainly affect your quality of life. So will your ability to access an adequate income and decent housing. And we have seen that fellow users are important. Since community care is more than the relations a user has with professionals, our global scale may paradoxically be a more sensitive measure of what users think of community care overall. This is because the question was phrased in terms of the *service*, not an individual or even a professional group. The question was, 'overall, how would you rate the community care services here in (site name)?'

More traditional instruments (see Appendix A) which measure satisfaction in terms of a professional group, or in terms of a service identified with a single professional, may be missing important information.

As explained in chapter 5, we conducted UFM in the KCW site in both 1997 and 1999. When the 1997 results were ready we presented them to the commissioners and then engaged in a feedback intervention. The feedback to the commissioners was used in a strategy document they produced. Our intervention was aimed at informing as many frontline staff as possible about our findings.

We did not feed back everything but concentrated on highly specific topics. The core questions we used were:

* the information questions on your mental health problem, the side effects of medication and community resources. Also, the information topic on the site visits;

* all the CPA questions;

* the question on crisis contacts;

* the questions on involvement at the level of individual care both in the community and in hospital.

(See Appendices C and D for a full list of questions.)

There were two main reasons for choosing these questions. First, the findings showed a low number of users answering these questions in the affirmative and there was therefore room for improvement. So, the commissioners and provider managers in particular were very concerned that only half the people interviewed knew who to contact in times of crisis. Secondly, the user group thought these findings important. For example, when we first presented the skeleton questionnaire, right at the beginning of the project, it included questions on the CPA. Most of the group were unaware of the CPA and when we explained it and what it was supposed to accomplish, they were quite angry that no professional had mentioned it to them. It came as no surprise to the group that most interviewees had not heard of the CPA either but they thought it was an issue that should be raised in the feedback to professionals.

Intervention – feeding back the results

The first part of the intervention involved feedback to the project advisory group made up of the health authority, provider managers and the voluntary sector. The managers were responsible for both inpatient and community care. This served the double function of informing the advisory group and refining the feedback for frontline workers.

Next, we held a feedback lunch organised by the health authority, the project co-ordinator and the user group. It was held on health authority premises and they also provided the food. There were posters round the walls with the main findings and personal accounts of interviewing by members of the user group. Seventy frontline staff and twenty users attended. A member of the user group chaired the meeting. The project co-ordinator then presented the basic findings and explained why we thought they were cause for concern. Two further members of the user group presented their experience of interviewing, focusing on the issues selected for feedback. The chair then facilitated questions and discussion.

The final part of the feedback consisted of individual visits to CMHTs. The project co-ordinator and one member of the user group visited approximately half the CMHTs in the health authority and explained our findings, how we had generated them and why we thought they were important.

As this was happening, the commissioners circulated a strategy document to a wide range of stakeholders. This included a section with targets based on our findings.

One of the aims of the monitoring in 1999 was to find out if this intensive feedback to staff was related to any changes in how users viewed community and hospital care services.

Findings

The percentages who felt well-informed about their mental health problem, the side effects of medication and community resources all increased whilst they remained the same for the other information questions. For mental health problems and the side effects of medication these increases were statistically significant. There were also qualitative increases in information on side effects and community resources in the site visits.

There were statistically significant increases in all the CPA questions except the general question on the CPA itself.

There was a statistically significant increase in the percentage that said they knew who to contact in times of crisis.

There was no significant increase in the proportion that felt involved in care planning and no discernible improvement in involvement during the site visits.

There were no significant increases or decreases on responses to questions that were not the subject of feedback.

Statistical details can be found in table AB.8 in Appendix B.

Comment

Most of the questions which were the subject of feedback showed a change over time whilst the questions which were not subject to feedback stayed constant. This is itself important because it gives us confidence in the validity of our method. The exception to this picture is involvement at the level of individual care.

What these findings suggest is that highly targeted, specific feedback can bring about change in the direction of greater responsiveness to the user. It may be more effective to use targeted, specific feedback like this rather than generalised arguments about user empowerment. This may be the reason the user involvement questions failed to show a difference. 'Involvement' is more abstract than 'information about..' and workers may have less idea how to bring it about. We would recommend that feedback consequent on the results of user monitoring should be as specific and concrete as possible. Other methods need to be used to bring about changes in more complex issues like user involvement.

Conclusion

The longitudinal study in KCW shows that it is possible to bring about change in users' experiences of hospital and community care services. Whilst the improvements must be largely the result of efforts on the part of purchasers, providers and frontline staff, the user-focused and targeted way it was done may have made the difference.

PART 3

SUMMING UP

Overview

In the following chapters, we draw out some of the main themes from the body of the report. We shall not try to cover everything but will focus on two main issues. These cross chapters which, we would argue, contain sufficient comment on the individual topics already.

Firstly, we will look at similarities and differences across and between sites.

Secondly, we will consider how the questions we have used in this research can be considered as a set of standards for good mental health services. This will include a discussion of whether the data we have presented can be used for benchmarking.

In chapter 5, we described the sites and the people interviewed. We saw that they varied widely in their social, ethnic, gender and geographical make-up. It might then have been predicted that the different projects would come up with a variety of findings in terms of how users perceived mental health and associated services. We did, indeed, find differences and in the expected directions. That is, where differences in responses were found they tended to favour the more affluent areas and not the deprived inner-city ones.

However, at first sight the picture from our findings is one of consistency of responses from the users interviewed. There are relatively few striking differences between the groups. Huntingdon provides talking treatments and this is welcome. Crises are not dealt with by the police in the county and users know a little more about CPA than those in the inner-city. However, Huntingdon users respond to questions about medication, information and involvement in the same way as users from KCW. The results of the overall satisfaction measure are remarkably consistent across sites.

We were slightly surprised by the level of consistency we discovered if only because the issue of resources is always argued to be so important in mental health care. The user movement, on the other hand, has always said that there is more to it than resources: that mental health care is to do with issues of attitudes, dignity, choice and respect.

Most of the people we interviewed were receiving rather a lot of mental health input. They almost all took medication, many went to day centres regularly and several lived in hostels or nursing homes. A significant proportion had recent hospital admissions and many were actually inpatients when we interviewed them. A lot of mental health input is what they had in common, however poor or affluent their community. It must be remembered that our samples in Huntingdon and Scarborough were very small compared to the large numbers we interviewed in inner London and that more research in rural sites is probably needed. However, we provisionally conclude that if you are somebody who makes, or is forced to make, heavy use of mental health services, you will have certain common experiences, whoever you are, wherever you go for care.

This is emphatically not to deny the differences and the exceptions. Beyond the level of intensive care units, security has its own logic. Women are plain scared in acute wards, never mind higher levels of security. It is not an accident that talking therapies are more widely available in the most middle-class site.

The most important difference, however, refers to ethnicity. We found relatively few differences on grounds of ethnicity *within* the groups in inner-London. But in these sites, users from black and minority ethnic communities were hugely over-represented in the first place. We had access to the census data on ethnic minorities in KCW and we found that black users are over-represented five-fold on the top tier of the CPA relative to their numbers in the local population. Everything we have said about KCW and Opendoor applies disproportionately to ethnic minority users.

How does a user get placed on the top tier of the CPA in the first place? A criterion used in KCW was the need for help from the full multi-disciplinary team. But this does not quite get to the bottom of it. People are deemed to need this help if they are vulnerable or at risk. This is not simply a diagnostic criterion; it is a social judgement. In a separate exercise for KCW, we showed that black users are more likely to be identified as at risk of violence to others than white users. So it could be argued that there are social stereotypes at work here and our findings are consistent with those reviewed in Fernando *et al.* (1998) as well as shedding some new light on what is going on.

Black users are more likely to find themselves on the top tier of the CPA to begin with and, once there, the quality of their experience will be different not least because they are identified as risky. We would still argue that once identified as candidates for the top tier of the CPA, users will have certain common experiences in addition to those on which they differ. For example, almost all the users we spoke to felt they were considered as less than fully competent by the mental health system.

Our experiences with our user-interviewers can shed some light on this. As we said in chapter 2, and is evident from the personal accounts in chapter 3, many people came to the groups convinced that they would not be able to participate or carry out the work. One way of putting this is to say that they had very low expectations of themselves. This is something the mental health system seems to promote. So, you do not give information or the opportunity to be involved to people not competent to understand it. There is a particular image of people with mental health problems in play in services and, of course, in society more generally. Black users have an additional image to contend with.

This may be overstating the case but there is a degree of consistency, as well as some clear differences, in our findings. The picture of mental health services gleaned from UFM may have some general relevance. It is not a particularly pretty picture and it has nevertheless to be set in the context of the fact that the services in which we carried out UFM may be amongst the most progressive in the country.

The core questions from the community schedules, which were reported on throughout Part 2, are reproduced in Appendix C. These questions were included in all six questionnaires with a few omissions. They were developed first by the KCW group and retained by the succeeding groups even while these groups dropped other questions and added new ones for their specific project and locale. The 61 users who were involved in the UFM projects took these core questions to be central for finding out about the key elements of contemporary community care. In this sense, the core questions can be considered as user-defined standards for good community care services. In parallel fashion, the questions for the site visits, reproduced at Appendix D, can be seen as user-defined standards for good acute care services.

In relation to the community questions, we also singled out a few areas for special consideration. Two factors led to the identification of these areas. First, that the percentage of users interviewed who had the element of care in place was low and second that those few who did have the element of care in place were happier with services overall than the rest. This sub-set of standards has been identified by analysing what the interviewees told us. It is a statistical analysis, explained in Part 2, and it has its limitations.

Focusing on this sub-set of standards does not detract from the importance of the core questions or standards as a whole. It is simply the outcome of a particular procedure based on data about low levels of care and associations with overall satisfaction. While the core questions for both community and acute services were arrived at by intensive discussion in the user groups, the sub-set of questions we will focus on here were arrived at by analysing the responses we collected from interviewing over 200 users who were living in the community and who had been identified as experiencing the most severe disabilities. It is their voice that has led us to focus on this sub-set of standards in this section of the report.

The sub-set of standards derived in this way can be divided into those which operate at a service level and those which pertain to individual care. There are three service-level standards and four individual ones. The final service-level dimension was not derived in the same statistical way as the others. It comes from what we were told about inpatient care both by those interviewed during the site visits and those who had recently experienced acute provision.

Service level

- Information on the full range of community care issues to be held by CMHTs.

- Information on the side effects of medication to be made available to all and at all sites which dispense medication.

- Alternatives to inpatient care and improvements in the units that remain.

Standards identified in this way look rather different to those which mental health services currently have to work to. These are the standards of the National Service Framework for Mental Health to which can be added proposals in the recently published NHS Plan.

The NSF standards do not mention information at all and yet we have seen how important this is in the difficult task of negotiating the agencies and resources involved in receiving mental health services and ensuring a good quality of life. Our user groups knew that it was important to ask about information and they included several information questions in the schedule. The people we interviewed showed us that access to sufficient information was related to overall satisfaction. Across three sites, every single information question was related to overall satisfaction.

Information was particularly important when it came to the side effects of medication. Branded prescriptions now contain leaflets on the side effects of medication. These should be available with prescriptions dispensed from hospital pharmacies and they should be available in inpatient facilities. Non-medical staff who take on the keyworking role, e.g. social workers, should have a basic knowledge of the side effects of the common psychotropic drugs. People isolated in the community, who never went out, with a home help doing their weekly shop and a CPN doing home visits, told us that they had insufficient information about the side effects of the depot injections they were receiving. This seems a very basic point to make but make it we must.

One proposal in the NSF that is in line with our findings is the endorsement of alternatives to hospital for some people in crisis. This is developed in the NHS Plan with the promise of universal access to crisis resolution teams. We are sure our informants would be pleased with this. At the same time, we have stressed that acute units will remain and it is likely that they will become services for the most distressed people, often those who are detained. They must not be allowed to deteriorate even further than their already appalling state. They need to be improved both environmentally and therapeutically.

Individual care

The sub-set of standards for individual care which we derived statistically are phrased as the specific questions were phrased, with appropriate grammatical transformations:

- needs assessment to take account of the user's strengths and abilities

- doctors to negotiate levels of medication with users

- users never to feel overmedicated

- users to be involved in care planning.

In discussing assessment of service users' needs, the NSF focuses on risk, problems and crises. There is no mention of taking into account service users' strengths and abilities and the positive aspects of their personalities and lives. Yet this specific issue was more significant to our users than general contentment with assessment. Most of them told us that their strengths were not taken into account when they were assessed but those who said they were scored higher on overall satisfaction than the rest. We did not ask about risk because our user groups did not raise it as an issue.

We saw in chapter 8 (Clinical Issues) that not all users thought that they were treated with respect and dignity when it came to medication. Discussing medication levels is one way of showing respect for a client. Ensuring that users do not feel overmedicated immeasurably increases their quality of life and ensures dignity. Overmedication can involve putting on a lot of weight, jerking, shuffling and dribbling. This is not dignified and it can lead to stigmatisation and social exclusion. Indeed, the visible effects of overmedication are a real problem for service users who know that these effects single them out as different.

The NSF promotes the prescription of atypical neuroleptics and SSRIs as these have fewer side effects. However, the *rationale* for this is greater engagement and greater compliance. The rationale for a standard says something about how it will be implemented. Moreover, the newer drugs have their own side effects such as sexual dysfunction.

Standard four of the NSF states that every service user should have a written copy of their care plan and, in the commentary, involvement in care planning is briefly mentioned. Our user groups thought these were important questions to ask *from the point of view of empowerment of service users*. Our informants were rarely involved in care planning but when they were this was significant in their overall perception of care. However, in the NSF user involvement is argued to be for reasons of sustaining engagement and not empowerment of service users. Using involvement to sustain engagement and bring about compliance means something different to involving people so that they can be empowered in the care process. It is the latter that our user groups intended when they asked about involvement.

Overall, our core questions from the community schedules represent standards for good practice in community health services. Similarly, the questions for the site visits represent standards for good practice in hospital provision. In the above paragraphs, we have considered a sub-set of the community standards which are important because the services they identify are available to only a small number of the users we interviewed and yet are associated with how users feel about the quality of care overall. This sub-set of standards has a particular resonance for people with the most severe mental health disabilities who are the group we interviewed. They are not often asked for their opinions about the care they receive. In most of our sites, the interviews were a novel experience for those who completed the questionnaire. It was critical to UFM that we reach such disabled users and it is their views that has led to the discussion of the sub-set of standards presented above.

Standards for mental health services that are carefully based on the user perspective look different to standards drawn up by professionals and civil servants. They are not a wish list. They have a firm evidence base. Their scope and rationale are user-based. We have distilled this information into a set of key recommendations which appear at the beginning of this report.

The value statement of the NSF emphasises respect, choice and dignity for the individual user. The NHS Plan is based on the premise that patients should be 'listened to' not 'talked at'. We share these values. But there may be a discrepancy between general values and specific standards as well as between general values and the rationales on which standards are based in government documents. The rationales of sustaining engagement and ensuring compliance sit uneasily with concepts of 'choice'. Overmedication is not consistent with dignity but it is consistent with the public safety agenda that underpins proposed reforms of the Mental Health Act. There is a tension at the heart of government policy on mental health between patient-centred services on the one hand and the public safety agenda, with its images of risk and incompetence, on the other.

If there is a rationale for our complete set of standards, it is the promotion of a 'strengths' and 'recovery' model of mental distress. In this context, we think the work reported here has provided a set of standards that could usefully complement those which are essentially service-led and profession-based even if we agree more with the values of the latter than their concrete content or their rationales. Our rationale comes down firmly on the side of the agenda of the NHS Plan and not on the side of those who promulgate the message that community care has failed and the public is at risk. One final message from those we interviewed was that however difficult life in the community might be at times, nobody wanted to go back to the old institutions and some of them had been there for years.

Benchmarking?

Having discussed the core questions, we may briefly consider the status of the data and whether it could be used for benchmarking. Benchmarking is the use of a set of standards, usually in statistical form, against which services can be assessed. Usually, benchmarking is against 'best practice' standards but it can be against the average. The aim is to adopt or improve on the benchmarks (Barnard, 1994). The question is whether the statistical data we have presented in previous chapters could be used as benchmarks for other mental health services.

As we have said repeatedly, the commissioners of UFM projects are not a randomly selected group. They wanted to evaluate their services from the user perspective and were prepared to try a user-focused method to do this. Most of them included a digest of our findings in strategy documents. 'Best practice' in terms of user satisfaction and user involvement might be expected from such a group and this would lead us to believe that our findings on our core questions represent benchmarks against which other services might be assessed.

Two things militate against such a conclusion. First, is the project co-ordinators' experience with frontline staff described in Part 1. Many were less than flattering about UFM or their clients' capacity to participate. There may a big difference between policy thrashed out at board meetings and practice on the ground. It is practice on the ground that matters to users.

Our second point is slightly different. 'Best practice' is a relative concept. The best that is available may still be poor absolutely. It may still be poor from the point of view of users. If our results represent best practice, or even just practice that is consistent everywhere, they are disappointing from the service user's point of view.

We therefore make two recommendations about the possible use of these results by other agencies:

- If the findings are to be used for benchmarking the aim should be to do better.
- The findings should be used as development as well as monitoring tools in order to improve response rates on the core questions in any agency which uses them.

Conclusion

The conclusion is simple. Mental health services need to change to become responsive to the expressed needs and demands of users and to respect their rights and responsibilities. We have shown that this is quite a generally applicable statement. In this chapter, we have tried to give some clear and simple pointers as to how this can be brought about. It requires a change of focus from a 'problems' to a 'strengths' model of service users. It should include user involvement at all levels from individual care, to local services, to national planning. In our work, we have tried to use UFM as a model of user involvement in the processes of research, monitoring and development. Doing this has enabled us to present a picture of contemporary community and hospital mental health services based wholly on the views of service users. This picture puts some new evidence and some new arguments into the mental health arena.

Evaluation and research can only do so much. It is up to others to take any information and any good ideas they find in this report forward. This is being done at the Sainsbury Centre, as the UFM team moves into development work and this will soon be made public. But we also hope that the locally flourishing user movement and associated decision-makers will use our findings and our ideas to promote user-focused services and user involvement in localities beyond those who participated in this report as well as at a national level.

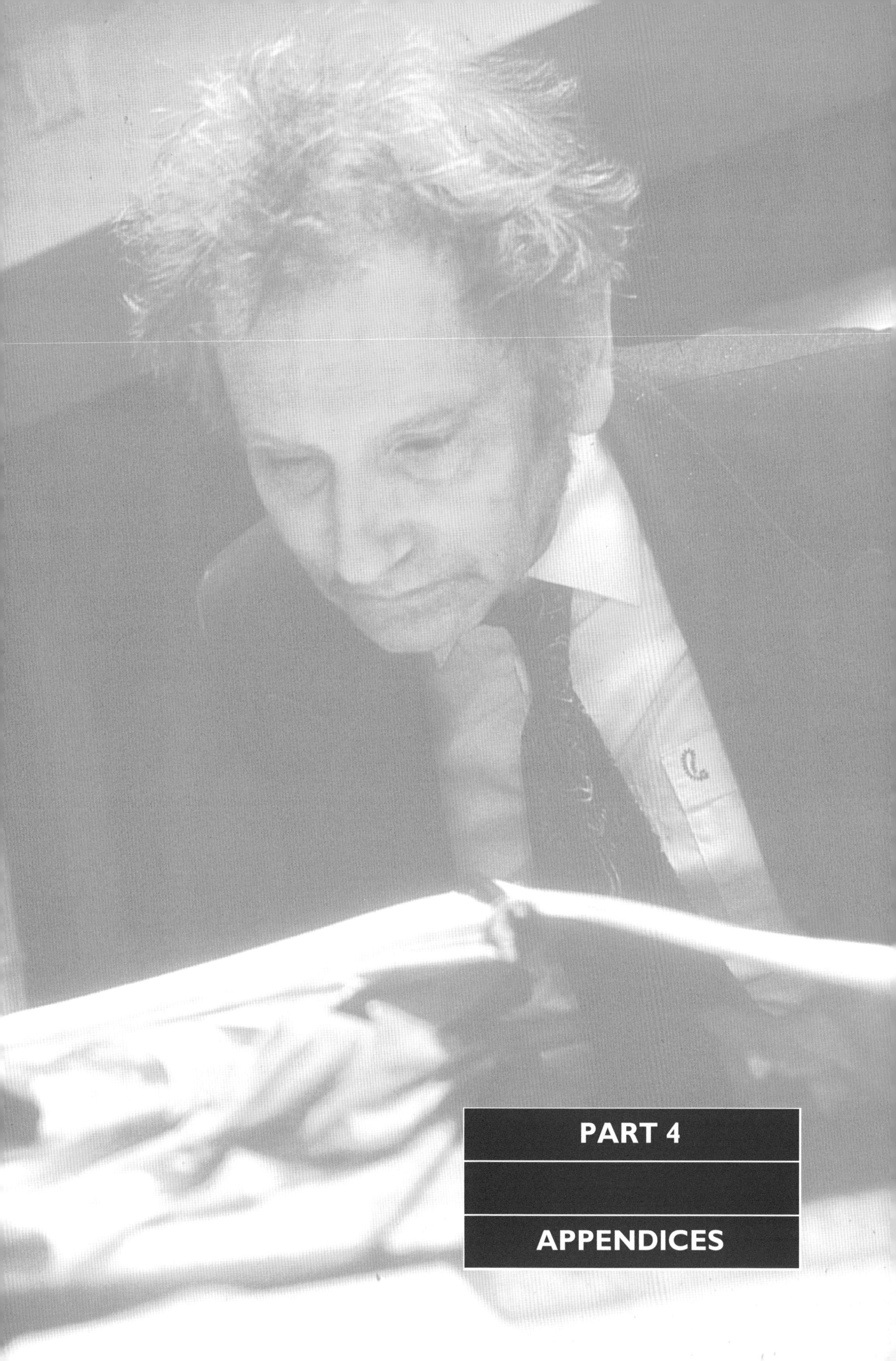

PART 4

APPENDICES

METHODOLOGY

This appendix considers UFM in relation to the more academic methodological issues. It is not for the general reader but for those interested in more technical methodological questions. We thought it important to include this appendix because we will try to show that UFM measures up well as a research technique in its own right and should not be considered to be methodologically 'soft' because it is user-focused.

We will proceed by relating UFM to issues raised in the literature on consumer satisfaction. As must be clear by now, a UFM interview schedule, or site visit workbook, is more than a tool for measuring consumer satisfaction. These instruments attempt to paint a picture of the details of community living for people with severe and enduring mental health problems. However, UFM instruments do contain satisfaction questions. And other questions in the schedules are strongly linked to satisfaction. Since there is considerable literature on user satisfaction in the field of mental health, it is appropriate to ask how UFM as a method is located in relation to the issues raised by that literature.

In order to make the discussion manageable, it is structured around some of the themes deployed by Stallard (1996) in his critique of the user satisfaction literature. Like Stallard, this discussion will concentrate on the UK literature except in respect of the issue of client versus professional interviewers. Literature published since Stallard's critique will be brought in where appropriate.

The topics to be considered are quantitative versus qualitative methodology and the design of questions, mental health service users as respondents, sampling, reliability and validity, one-off studies as opposed to cross-sectional or longitudinal studies and consumer versus professional interviewers.

Quantitative or qualitative?

There now exist a number of quantitative consumer satisfaction scales that have been used in the field of mental health. The Larsen Satisfaction Scale (Larsen *et al.* 1979) is an example. Typically they consist of a limited number of likert-type items and result in numerical scores. These are the kinds of satisfaction scales commented upon in chapter 12.

Recently, several commentators have criticised these sorts of scales. Crawford and Kessel (1999) argue that they are modelled on the measuring instruments of biomedical psychiatry, as if satisfaction were a 'thing', and ignore the complexity of users' feelings about the treatment they receive. Crawford and Kessel propose that qualitative methods give a more accurate picture. This call for more qualitative methods was also made by Stallard (1996) and has since been echoed by Greenwood et al. (1999) who found quantitative methods to be inadequate in their study of consumer satisfaction with inpatient facilities.

Probably the first survey to use a mix of quantitative and qualitative questions in the UK was the People First survey carried out by MIND (*Experiencing Psychiatry: Users' Views of Services,* Rogers, Pilgrim and Lacey, 1993). Crawford and Kessel take this study as a litmus test because it showed far lower satisfaction with mental health services than had been found with the quantitative scales. Indeed, earlier work with the standardised instruments had found satisfaction running at around 90% and these findings were, for some, counter-intuitive. The current state of opinion, then, seems to be that open-ended qualitative questions are to be preferred over closed, quantitative questions.

Where is UFM located in this debate? A typical UFM questionnaire contains both closed questions and qualitative, open-ended questions. We would argue that there is a good rationale for closed questions *as long as they are user-defined*. It is the local UFM user-group who decides the questions that make up an interview schedule. They are asked to frame questions according to their own experience of what is important in the community or hospital care process.

Stallard argues that focus groups are a good method of generating questions. Our method is quite close to this except that it is extended over time with several opportunities for the refinement of questions.

UFM questionnaires are very different to those designed by mental health professionals and certainly very different to the quantitative scales discussed above. To take just one example, satisfaction with your psychiatrist. A quantitative scale will attempt to 'measure' this with a likert-type item. UFM questionnaires also have a straightforward satisfaction question but, in addition, they ask about choice and influence, whether the psychiatrist negotiates medication and whether strengths and abilities are taken into account in the assessment process. Obviously, these are not direct satisfaction questions. We have seen that they do show strong associations with global measures of satisfaction. We do not think this is because the two types of questions are measuring the 'same thing'. Rather, the discrete questions tap the detail of what makes for satisfaction.

The questions from UFM questionnaires listed above are 'closed' and the data quantitative. But because they have come from the users' perspective they allow issues to appear in the data, which are ignored by more orthodox measuring instruments. For UFM, then, it is perfectly appropriate to include a mix of closed and open questions in an interview schedule because the entire process is user-defined. It is also important that the closed questions are sufficiently specific and that they cover a range of issues.

Perhaps a final comparison will illustrate the point. Recently, the Mental Health Foundation (2000a) published its *Strategies for Living* report. The method used was qualitative following topic-based, in-depth interviewing. In other respects, the method was similar to UFM. The interviewers were users. The report argues that the method used is the only way to get detailed, rich information. This seems to be the current consensus. We would dispute it.

For example, both reports present data on users' views on medication. As has been seen in our report, the UFM data is statistical. The data from the Mental Health Foundation consists of selected verbatim quotes. However, both reports also contain interpretations of their data. And the interesting point is that these interpretations give very similar pictures of being a mental health service user on psychotropic medication. We conclude that the overall process in user-led research is more important than any specific method. Naturally, we also think there are advantages to closed questions and some statistical presentation of results. It was statistical analysis that enabled us to focus on a sub-set of the user-focused standards we proposed for a good mental health service. This is not to deny the validity of qualitative methods. Rather, it is an argument for methodological pluralism.

Mental health service users as respondents

In the early days of consumer satisfaction studies in the field of mental health, questions were raised as to whether service users were mentally capable of filling in the scales in a rational way (Carlsmith and Aronson, 1963). Again, the finding of very high satisfaction ratings with the quantitative scales was raised. Langs (1976), in a psychoanalytic paper, proposed that these high ratings were due to transference (see also Lebow, 1983). It should be noted here that the unusually high ratings are being analysed in terms of patient characteristics rather than looking to problems with the measuring instruments themselves.

The early scepticism about the mental capacity of mental health service users has given way, in the research literature at least, to an acceptance that service users can make valid and sound judgements about the services that they receive. It is accepted that these judgements can and should influence the care delivery process.

However, in doing UFM we have experienced scepticism amongst professionals about the mental capacity of people with severe and enduring mental illness to answer our questionnaires. On one occasion, an interpreter, himself a mental health professional, refused to do the interview on the grounds that the interviewee was too young and too sick. A psychotherapist said of one client, "you can't interview that woman. Her criticisms of services are a symptom of her mental illness".

In our research, where we have talked with over 500 service users, there has been only one occasion where the interview was rendered impossible by the mental state of the user. This user insisted on being interviewed on the toilet wearing only a jumper and he was not able to concentrate on the questions. The body of this report is testament to the capacity of mental health service users to make sound, valid and helpful judgements and comments on the services they receive.

Sampling

UFM uses random sampling. This is not only in order to do statistical analysis but also to gather a broad range of views. We seek to include people who would never volunteer to be interviewed, for instance those who are housebound or in other ways isolated. Isolated people do not frequent the kinds of places, such as day centres or community centres, where researchers often find their subjects. Random sampling ensures they will be included.

Random sampling can be time consuming because of the importance of confidentiality. Some authorities are prepared to release names, for instance all those on the top tier of the CPA, but others are concerned about confidentiality. Then it is a question of the authorities assigning numbers to names, the random sampling being done on the numbers, and the authorities contacting the selected interviewees. UFM is prepared for this complexity because we would like our samples to be as representative as possible.

Stallard noted that response rates for community samples in mental health are typically very low. He cites one study where the response rate was 13%. Inpatient satisfaction surveys (e.g. Greenfield et al., 1999) usually have much higher response rates. This is because they are dealing with a captive population. There are many reasons why response rates from community samples may be low. People may have moved or be homeless. They may not fully understand the letter they have received. They may not have the time to do an interview. Stallard makes the argument that it is important to be sure that non-respondents do not differ in significant ways from respondents.

UFM, in its work with community samples, typically has response rates of about 30%. The question then arises whether the samples are biased in the sense of there being a systematic difference between those who we interview and those who we do not. For instance, keyworkers might have passed the letters on or not in a selective way. If this were so, the statistics done in this report would be invalid.

Because of other work we were doing for the health authority in KCW we had a database with demographic and clinical information on all those on the top tier of the CPA. Demographic comparisons were then made between those who agreed to be interviewed and the total CPA population. In these cases, we found no differences on the demographic variables. We did not, for example, find a lower response rate from users from black and ethnic minority communities as might be expected given these communities suspicion of mental health services. Of course, the group interviewed may still have been unrepresentative in their opinions of community care services. To find this out is beyond the scope of UFM. It is beyond the scope of nearly all social research to establish representativeness on the dependent variable and it is a limitation.

Reliability and validity

Stallard argues that greater effort should be expended on standardising instruments and establishing their reliability and validity. However, a UFM questionnaire or site visiting workbook is not a psychometric instrument. It is not even clear that they ever could be. To insist on this would be to commit the biomedical fallacy (Crawford and Kessel, 1999). This is not unusual in the consumer satisfaction field.

Let us look at this notion of the 'biomedical fallacy' in a little more detail. It has long been argued in the sociological and psychological literature (Cicourel, 1964; Harre and Secord, 1972) that 'measuring' an opinion is not like measuring a physical quality. This is because measuring instruments in the physical sciences do not affect the property they are measuring. For instance, a thermometer cannot affect the temperature of the water it is taking. However, the administration of a satisfaction scale is a piece of social interaction and the scale and the person who administers it will have an effect on the response that is made. In this sense the property being measured is reactive. Unlike the water, it is affected by the measuring instrument and the context of administration. Attitudes and opinions are not invariant qualities.

Cicourel (1964) argues that it is fruitless to try to minimise the social qualities of the interaction. For example, attempts to use only one trained interviewer who is 'standardised' across all the interviews will fail because the quality of the interaction will differ according to social characteristics of the interviewee. This problem is recognised in the more orthodox literature as the problem of 'matching' interviewer and interviewee on characteristics such as gender, social class and ethnicity. This is a practice we follow ourselves. However, we also go some way with Cicourel's argument that the essentially social and reactive nature of psychological and social measuring instruments can never be neutralised.

So what is to be done? One answer is simple although it is also partial. That is, to be as explicit as possible about the methodology used so that it is transparent to the reader who can then judge for themselves its strengths and limitations. We hope we have fulfilled this condition in this report.

The other answer is to *capitalise* on the essentially social qualities of the instrument and the interview context. This is what is done with UFM. The questions arise out of social interaction between users. The interviewers openly share their experience of psychiatric services with interviewees and they rely on shared experience and empathy. We believe this goes beyond the 'good rapport' counselled of traditional interviewers. Moreover, the analyses are carried out by users (the project co-ordinators) who interpret the figures resulting from the interviews from a user's perspective. We hope this is evident throughout this report.

It should now be clear why Stallard's plea for test-re-test reliability would not make sense for a UFM instrument (actually, we do not think it makes sense for any social instrument). The interview itself is designed to make users think, in a way that they perhaps have not done before, about the services they receive and their own choice and empowerment. The carrying out of the interview can itself influence the way the user thinks about the services they receive so one would not expect the same responses to the same interview schedule, say two months later. The experience of responding to the first schedule and the first interview means that the interviewee will react to the second situation with altered eyes. Because of this they will give different responses and so the method would appear 'unreliable'.

There is one problem of reliability that UFM must nevertheless address. Typically, a UFM project uses six to eight interviewers. How do we know that they are all implementing the questionnaire or site visit workbook in the same way? Logistically, and for the reasons given in the last paragraph, they cannot all be asked to interview the same person to see if they all get the same results. It is well known that the more thorough the training of a group of interviewers the higher the inter-rater reliability. For example, Roncone *et al.* (1999) were able to increase the level of inter-rater reliability amongst a group of clinically inexperienced assessors on the BPRS to the same level as that for experienced assessors by the simple expedient of training them. We showed in chapter 2 that our groups of interviewers receive thorough training.

What of validity? The establishment of external validity is impossible and probably nonsensical. What would be the external criterion of satisfaction with community care services in mental health? One suggestion has been staying engaged with services. But there are all kinds of reasons why people may drop out of services and lack of satisfaction is only one of them. Indeed, reasons may be positive as Stallard himself acknowledges. In any event, professionals often go to great lengths to stop users 'disengaging' and they have the ultimate sanction of compulsory detention. In this situation, asking users about their satisfaction is a far better measure than any other 'external' criterion.

UFM questionnaires (but not site visit workbooks) can establish construct validity. We have seen that the global measure of satisfaction is statistically significantly associated with discrete questions about the provision of information, needs assessment and the experience of taking medication. It also correlates with the degree to which people see themselves as involved in their care. These are the discrete questions we predicted would be associated with overall satisfaction (see Appendix B).

One-off studies, cross-sectional studies and longitudinal studies

Stallard criticises consumer satisfaction research in mental health in the UK as characterised by one-off studies, each constructing their own instruments, which do not follow through their work and therefore can have no influence on the planning process. This last point is important for UFM. The technique was always meant to influence planners and managers in the direction of more user-sensitive services and was never meant as a purely research endeavour.

We would argue that UFM, as we have been carrying it out for the last four years, meets Stallard's points. UFM has been carried out in eight sites, six of them employing community questionnaires with common core questions. Although the questionnaire was tailored by each UFM group to its particular emphases on community care and the particular project it was asked to do, the structure remains constant and some core questions are asked in each of the six projects.

We carried out one longitudinal study. We found that user satisfaction with community care services changed as a result of policies implemented consequent upon feedback from the UFM team.

Consumer versus professional interviewers

In this appendix, we have already had occasion to comment on the early findings of very high satisfaction ratings evinced by mental health service consumers. One response to this 'halo effect', as we have seen, was to analyse it in terms of patient characteristics. More recently, it has been seen as a function of the instruments used to measure satisfaction.

An alternative response, now evident in the North American literature (Polowycz et al., 1993; Clark et al. 1999) is to explain the high satisfaction ratings in terms of interviewer characteristics. These authors argue that high satisfaction ratings are a result of the interview being conducted by mental health professionals. At the extreme, satisfaction interviews are carried out by the professional who is providing the service which is being assessed. It is argued that users would be unwilling to criticise such services in case there were repercussions, even loss of the service. But even where an independent mental health professional carried out the interview, users might be worried that critical responses would be relayed back to the service provider. It is therefore proposed that user interviewers might gain more valid responses.

The authors cited above have therefore carried out studies, using randomised designs, comparing responses to professional interviewers with responses to client interviewers. These studies show that users are more likely to make critical comments to client interviewers than they are to professional interviewers. It should be noted that the instruments used in these studies were standardised ones with established reliability scores. Yet there was a systematic difference between client and professional interviewers. This is also further evidence of the instability of reliability in social research.

The deployment of user interviewers is central to UFM as a method. We have always argued that user interviewers gain a more valid picture of using community care and hospital services, and satisfaction with those services, than professional interviewers. In addition to the design of the above studies, of course, we also deployed user-defined instruments so that the content of the interview, as well as the person who carried it out, provide an enabling social context for the interviewee.

Has UFM overcome the 'halo' effect? On our global satisfaction scale, average ratings tend to cluster just above the mid-point. This finding is highly consistent across six sites and seems more realistic than ratings of 90%. It also shows considerable room for improvement in services.

Conclusion

In this appendix, we have argued the more academic aspects of methodology. In chapter 2 we described the process of doing UFM and we did this in narrative form. To the experienced and more academic researcher it may have looked like a very 'soft' process. Here we have taken on some of the 'hard' issues and hope to have shown that UFM is a well thought-through, rigorous and robust method. There is no contradiction between involving users and high standards of research.

The statistic used in this appendix is 'student's t' which assessed the difference between people who answered 'yes' and people who answered 'no' on key questions in terms of how they scored on the overall satisfaction score.

Only significant results are reported. It was decided that results would be reported if a test was found to be significant on at least two sites. The variables reported were tested on all sites where the questions were asked. Therefore results not reported are also not significant for those sites. Usually differences were in the expected direction but small numbers were involved. In some cases independent variables were very skewed with only one or two people endorsing a question thus making the t test meaningless.

The results reported below come from hypothesis tests. We did not test every single relationship thereby increasing the likelihood of chance significance findings. Where a test was carried out and no significant relationship found, this is reported in the text.

Information provision (see chapter 6)

Table AB.1 Differences in overall satisfaction according to whether users had sufficient information on a range of issues in Scarborough				
	Mean difference	T	Df	P
Mental health problem	2.38	2.95	32	0.006
Side effects	1.73	2.05	28	0.05
Housing	1.8	1.95	12	0.074
Benefits	3.15	4.22	23	0.000
Work	2.03	2.42	29	0.022
Community resources	2.08	2.63	28	0.014

Df = Degrees of freedom   P = Probability value

Table AB.2	Differences in overall satisfaction according to whether users had sufficient information on a range of issues in KCW I			
	Mean difference	T	Df	P
Mental health problem	2.56	3.98	35.88	0.000
Side effects	1.25	1.96	45.26	0.056
Housing	2.48	3.66	44	0.001
Benefits	1.01	1.22	45	0.22
Work	0.40	0.569	55	0.55
Community resources	2.11	3.39	49	0.001

Table AB.3	Differences in overall satisfaction according to whether users had sufficient information on a range of issues in KCW II			
	Mean difference	T	Df	P
Mental health problem	2.57	3.98	35.89	0.000
Side effects	2.45	3.83	62	0.000
Housing	2.64	4.33	58	0.000
Benefits	1.93	2.51	58	0.015
Work	0.8	1.33	73	0.187
Community resources	2.54	4.44	62	0.000

Assessment (see chapter 8 – Clinical Issues)

Strengths and abilities

Table AB.4	Differences in overall satisfaction according to whether users felt their strengths and abilities had been taken into account when their needs were assessed			
	Mean difference	T	Df	P
Opendoor CSS	2.64	2.59	17	0.019
Huntingdon	2.57	2.71	15	0.016
Scarborough	2.65	2.61	21	0.016
KCW I	1.44	2.11	54	0.04
KCW II	2.04	3.40	66	0.001

Treatment (see chapter 8 – Clinical Issues)

Medication

Table AB.5	Differences in overall satisfaction according to whether users reported that their consultant negotiated medication levels with them			
	Mean difference	T	df	P
KCW I	1.85	2.57	51	0.013
KCW II	2.4	3.73	67	0.000

Table AB.6	Differences in overall satisfaction according to whether users reported that they felt overmedicated			
	Mean difference	T	Df	P
KCW I	2.38	3.78	50	0.000
KCW II	2.71	4.66	65	0.000

User involvement (see chapter 10)

Table AB.7	Differences in overall satisfaction according to whether users reported being involved in drawing up their care plan			
	Mean difference	T	Df	P
Opendoor CSS	3.98	2.97	17	0.009
Huntingdon	1.6	2.36	18	0.029
KCW I	0.91	2.02	36	0.05
KCW II	2.00	2.54	47	0.014

KCW longitudinal (see chapter 13 – KCW Over Time)

Table AB.8 gives Chi-Square and associated p values for contingency tables drawn up on the basis of 'before' and 'after' responses to all the questions highlighted in the feedback intervention in KCW (chapter 13). In this case, we are reporting non-significant as well as significant results. Degrees of freedom were 1 in all cases. Percentages for KCW I and KCW II can be found in the body of the report.

Table AB.8 Chi-Square and p values testing the difference between proportions at two points in time for a range of variables in KCW		
	Chi-Square	P >
Information about mental health problem	4.0	0.05
Information about side effects of medication	9.6	0.001
Information about community resources	> 0	Ns
Aware of CPA	3.24	Ns
Knows who keyworker is	14.11	0.001
Has care plan	6.21	0.025
Knows date of next CPA review	8.34	0.005
Involved in drawing up care plan	> 0	Ns
Knows who to contact in a crisis	10.95	0.001

CORE QUESTIONS FROM THE
COMMUNITY INTERVIEWS

This Appendix lists the core questions used in the one-to-one community interviews which were reported on in Part 2 of this report. The core questions were developed by the first KCW project and they were retained by further UFM projects as other questions were dropped and new ones added by each individual project. The core questions are listed in the order in which they appear in Part 2 rather than the order in which they were asked during the interviews.

1   Do you have enough information about your mental health problem?

2   Do you have enough information about the side effects of any medication you are taking?

3   Do you have sufficient information about issues relating to your housing?

4   Do you have sufficient information about your benefits?

5   Do you have enough information about work schemes available locally?

6   Do you have enough information about local community groups and resources?

7   Do you know what CPA is all about and what it is for?

8   Do you have a CPA keyworker?

9   Do you have a care plan?

10   Do you know the date of your next CPA review?

11   Do you think your needs have been properly assessed?

12   When you were assessed, were your strengths and abilities taken into account as well as your problems?

13   Do you take medication for your mental health difficulties?

14   Do you take the medication by mouth or by injection?

15   Does your consultant negotiate your medication levels with you?

16   Do you think the medication helps you?

17   If you are given an injection, is it given with dignity and respect for you?

18   Do you experience side effects from your medication?

19   How distressing for you are these side effects (on a scale from 1 to 5)?

20   Do you feel over medicated at all?

21   Do you have sufficient access to talking therapies?

22   How satisfied are you with the talking therapies you receive?

23   Do you know who to contact when you are experiencing a crisis?

24   Do you have a relapse plan?

25   Have you been in hospital in the last year?

26 Was your discharge managed well?

27 Were you involved in planning your discharge?

28 Have you been detained in hospital under the Mental Health Act (sectioned) in the past year?

29 Were your rights under the Mental Health Act properly explained to you?

30 Were you offered the services of an advocate?

31 What types of help would you like if you experienced a crisis in the future:
   - Face-to-face contact with a professional?
   - Telephone contact with a professional?
   - Advice about medication?
   - Non-medical forms of help such as a crisis house?
   - GP backup?

32 Have you ever had contact with the police because of your mental health problem?

33 Did you find the police helpful?

34 Did the police officers treat you with dignity and respect?

35 Did you think that the police used unnecessary force with you?

36 Are you involved in drawing up your care plan?

37 Are you involved in setting up your CPA reviews?

38 Are you involved in running any day centres or work projects you attend?

39 Do you know about user groups in your community?

40 How influential do you think these groups are?

41 Do you find other users helpful?

42 Do you know what an advocate is?

43 Have you ever used one?

44 How satisfied were you with the advocacy service provided to you?

45 Do you know that you have the right to see the records kept about you?

46 Have you ever seen them?

47 Would you feel able to make a complaint if you felt it was necessary?

48 Have you ever made a complaint about health or social services (or Opendoor for Opendoor clients)?

49 If not, what stopped you?

50 If so, how satisfied were you with the outcome?

51 How satisfied are you with your keyworker?

52 How satisfied are you with your consultant psychiatrist?

53 How satisfied are you with the junior doctors you see?

54 How satisfied are you with your CPN?

55 How satisfied are you with your social worker?

56 How satisfied are you with your community support worker?

57 To finish with, here is a scale from 1 to 10. 1 means terrible and 10 means excellent. Overall, how would you rate the community mental health services you receive?

1   Is the location of the service convenient for the people who use it?

2   Is the service easy and safe to get to and from?

3   Is it a safe place to attend as an inpatient?

4   Are there too many rules and regulations?

5   Is it possible to get a drink whenever one is wanted or needed?

6   Is there a café?

7   Do the staff have warm and respectful professional relationships with the patients?

8   Are treatments used by the service safe and effective?

9   Does the service provide a range of alternative and complementary therapies?

10 Does the service provide a range of talking therapies such as group therapy and individual counselling?

11 Does the service provide interesting and beneficial activities during the day?

12 Does the service provide interesting and beneficial activities at evenings and weekends?

13 Does the service provide a variety of quiet, relaxing TV and radio-free areas?

14 Does the service provide a variety of No Smoking areas including quiet rooms and the TV lounge?

15 Does the service enable visiting at any time?

16 Does the service provide facilities for children to visit?

17 Is the service an attractive, clean and comfortable place to be in?

18 Are the toilets and bathrooms clean?

19 Is the kitchen open 24 hours per day?

20 Does the service provide access to pleasant areas outdoors?

21 Is sleeping accommodation provided in single rooms with TV and radio points?

22 Does the service provide separate, private bathing and washing facilities for men and for women?

23 Does the service provide separate, private sleeping facilities for men and for women?

24 Does the service provide facilities to meet religious and spiritual needs?

25 Does the service provide well-prepared and nutritious food, taking account of personal preferences, religious or spiritual needs?

26 Does the service provide facilities for exercise?

27 Can you get independent advocacy if you need it?

28 Do people get all the information they need about their treatment and care?

29 Are people involved enough in decisions about their care and treatments?

30 Is there a patients' council for this service?

REFERENCES

Barnes, M. (1997) *Care, Communities and Citizens*. London and New York: Longman.

Barnard, J. (1994) Benchmarking in the service sector. *Organisation Development Journal*, **12** (4) 65-72.

Bauer, M., Gaskell, G. & Allum, N. (2000) Quality, quantity and knowledge interests: avoiding confusion. In M. Bauer and G. Gaskell (eds) *Qualitative Researching with Text, Image and Sound*. London: Sage.

Biehal, N., Marsh, P. & Fisher, M. (1992) Rights and social work. In Coote, A. (ed) *The Welfare of Citizens*. London: IPPR/River Oram Press.

Campbell, P. (1996) The history of the user movement in the United Kingdom. In T. Heller, J. Reynolds, R. Gomm, R. Muston and S. Pattison (eds) *Mental Health Matters. A Reader*. Milton Keynes: The Open University.

Carlsmith, M.J. & Aronson, E. (1963) Some hedonic consequences of the confirmation of expectancies. *Journal of Abnormal and Social Psychology*, **66**, 151-156.

Cicourel, A. (1964) *Method and Measurement in Sociology*. Illinois: Glencoe Free Press.

Clark C.C., Scott, E.A., Boydell, K.M. & Goering P (1999) Effects of client interviewers on client-reported satisfaction with mental health services. *Psychiatric Services*, **50** (7) 961-963.

Crawford, M.J. & Kessel, A.S. (1999) Not listening to patients – the use and misuse of patient satisfaction studies. *International Journal of Social Psychiatry*, **45** (1) 1-6.

Department of Health (1990a) *NHS and Community Care Act*. London: HMSO.

Department of Health (1990b) *Access to Health Records Act*. London: HMSO.

Department of Health (1995) *Building Bridges*. London: HMSO.

Department of Health (1999a) *National Service Framework for Mental Health*. London: The Stationery Office.

Department of Health (1999b) *Safer Services: Confidential Inquiry into Homicides and Suicides by Mentally Ill People*. London: The Stationery Office.

Department of Health (2000). *The NHS Plan*. London: The Stationery Office.

Fernando, S., Ndegwa, D. and Wilson, M. (eds) (1998) *Forensic Psychiatry, Race and Culture*. London: Routledge.

Good Practices in Mental Health (1989) *Treated Well?... ... ...* by Camden Mental Health Consortium. London: GPMH.

Greenwood, N., Key A., Burns, T. *et al.* (1999) Satisfaction with inpatient psychiatric services. Relationship to patient and treatment factors. *British Journal of Psychiatry*, **174**, 159-163.

Jamdagni, L. (1996) *Purchasing for Black Populations*. London: King's Fund.

Kemp, R., Hayward, P., Applewhaite, G. *et al.* (1996) Compliance therapy in psychotic patients: randomised controlled trial. *British Medical Journal*, **312**, 345-349.

Jha, A., Bernadt, M., Brown, K., Sawicka, E. & Stein, G. (1998) Access to health records: psychiatric patients and patients with diabetes compared. *Psychiatric Bulletin*, **22**, 309-312.

Harre, R. & Secord, P. (1972) *The Explanation of Social Behaviour*. Oxford: Blackwell.

Langs, R. (1976) *The bipersonal field*. New York: Jason Aronson.

Larsen, D.L., Attkinson, C.C., Hargreaves, A.A. *et al.* (1979) Assessment of client/patient satisfaction: development of a general scale. *Evaluation and Program Planning*, **2**,197-207.

Lebow, J.L. (1983) Research assessing consumer satisfaction with mental health treatment: a review of findings. *Evaluation and Program Planning*, **6**, 211-236.

Mental Health Foundation (2000a) *Strategies for Living*. London: MHF.

Mental Health Foundation (2000b) *Pull Yourself Together*. London: MHF.

Mental Health Task Force User Group (n.d.) *Advocacy: A Code of Practice*. London: NHSE.

Ndegwa, D. (1998) Clinical issues. In: Fernando, S., Ndegwa, D. and Wilson, M. (eds) *Forensic Psychiatry, Race and Culture*. London: Routledge.

Perkins, R. & Repper, J. (1998) *Dilemmas in Community Mental Health Practice: Choice or Control?* Oxford: Radcliffe Medical Press.

Polowycz, D., Brutus, M., Orvietto, B.S., Vidal, J. & Cipriana, D. (1993) Comparison of patient and staff surveys of consumer satisfaction. *Hospital and Community Psychiatry*, **44** (6) 589-691.

Read, J. and Wallcraft, J (1992) *Guidelines for Empowering Users of Mental Health Services*. London: Confederation of Health Service Employees and MIND.

Rogers, A., Pilgrim, D. & Lacey, R. (1993) *Experiencing Psychiatry: Users' Views of Services*. London: Macmillan and MIND.

Roncone, R., Ventura, J., Impallomeni, M., Falloon, I.R.H., Morosini, P.L., Chairavalle, E., & Cassacchia, M. (1999) Reliability of an Italian standardized and expanded Brief Psychiatric Rating Scale (BPRS 4.0) in raters with high vs. low clinical experience. *Acta Psychiatrica Scandinavica*, **100** (3) 229-236.

Rose, D. (1996) *Living in the Community*. London: SCMH.

Rose, D., Warner, L. & Ford, R. (submitted) The care and treatment of detained patients from black and minority ethnic communities.

Rose, D., Ford, R., Gawith, L., Lindley, P. and the KCW UFM User Group (1998) *In Our Expereince: User-Focused Monitoring of Mental Health Services in KCW HA*. London: SCMH.

The Sainsbury Centre for Mental Health (1998a) *Acute Problems*. London: SCMH.

The Sainsbury Centre for Mental Health (1998b) *Open All Hours*. London: SCMH.

The Sainsbury Centre for Mental Health (2000) *Taking Your Partners*. London: SCMH.

Stallard, P. (1996) The role and use of consumer satisfaction surveys in mental health services. *Journal of Mental Health*, **5** (4) 333-348.